Making a Difference!

For Youth with Cognitive Impairments

FIFTH EDITION

FACILITATOR CURRICULUM

An Adaptation of an Evidence-Based, Abstinence Approach to Teen Pregnancy and HIV/STD Prevention

Loretta Sweet Jemmott, PhD, RN, FAAN
John B. Jemmott, III, PhD
Konstance A. McCaffree, PhD, CSE
Regina Firpo-Triplett, MPH, CNC, MCHES
Brittany Louise-Hoffman Lucas, MPH, CHES

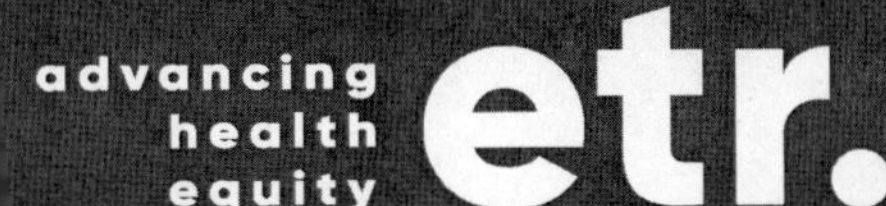

Published by ETR, 100 Enterprise Way, Suite G300, Scotts Valley, CA 95066-3248.

Printed in the United States of America.

Title No. A461

ISBN 978-1-56240-204-4

The original *Making a Difference* curriculum was developed, pilot-tested, implemented, and evaluated in a study funded by the National Institute of Mental Health (R01-MH52035).

This adaptation of *Making a Difference for Youth with Cognitive Impairments* was made possible by Funding Opportunity Number HHS-2016-ACF-ACYF-SR-1197 from the Department of Health and Human Services, Administration for Children and Families. Its contents are solely the responsibility of Kent Intermediate School District, dfusion and ETR and do not necessarily represent the official views of the Department of Health and Human Services, Administration for Children and Families.

18-1024

ETR End User License Agreement

PLEASE READ THIS AGREEMENT CAREFULLY. THIS END USER LICENSE AGREEMENT ("AGREEMENT") IS BETWEEN EDUCATION TRAINING AND RESEARCH ASSOCIATES, INC. (THE "COMPANY") AND THE PERSON/ORGANIZATION WHO PURCHASES / OPENS THIS PACKAGE OR USES THE MATERIAL WHICH ACCOMPANIES THIS AGREEMENT (THE "USER"). THIS AGREEMENT GIVES A USER THE RIGHT TO ACCESS AND USE THE COMPANY'S PRODUCTS AND SERVICES ("PRODUCTS") **LICENSED** FROM THE COMPANY PURSUANT TO A LICENSE AGREEMENT, CONTRACT, SALES OR PURCHASE ORDER, INVOICE OR CREDIT CARD PURCHASE ("LICENSE CONTRACT"). THE COMPANY IS WILLING TO GRANT A USER THE RIGHT TO ACCESS AND USE THE COMPANY'S PRODUCTS ONLY IF THE USER ACCEPTS ALL OF THE TERMS OF THIS AGREEMENT, AND PAYS OR HAS PAID THE COMPANY THE FULL PRICE (TO INCLUDE ALL APPLICABLE TAXES AND FEES) PURSUANT TO THE LICENSE CONTRACT. BY PURCHASING THE PRODUCTS AND AGREEING BY SIGNATURE, BY USE OF PRODUCTS OR BY "CLICK THROUGH" THE USER ACKNOWLEDGES THAT USER HAS READ THIS AGREEMENT, UNDERSTANDS IT, AND AGREES TO BE BOUND BY IT. IF THE USER DOES NOT AGREE TO ALL OF THE TERMS IN THIS AGREEMENT, THE USER SHOULD NOT ACCESS OR OTHERWISE UTILIZE THE PRODUCTS BECAUSE NO LICENSE SHALL HAVE BEEN GRANTED THERETO.

1. LICENSE. In consideration of the payment of the amount agreed to in the License Agreement Contract for the right to use Company's Products, and the User's adherence to all provisions of this Agreement, the Company grants the User a personal, non-exclusive, non-transferable license to access and use the Company's Products covered hereunder for educational purposes described in the License Agreement Contract in the United States of America, its territories and possessions.

2. RESTRICTIONS. User may not use, copy, modify or transfer the Products to others, in whole or in part, except as expressly provided in this Agreement. User may not create a derivative work based on the Products. The Products contain trade secrets and method patents of the Company, and the User may not reverse engineer, disassemble, decompile, adapt, modify or translate the Products, or otherwise attempt to derive its source code or the source code through which the Products is accessed, or authorize any third-party to do any of the foregoing. The license granted hereunder is personal to the User, and any attempt by the User to transfer any of the rights, duties or obligations hereunder shall terminate this Agreement and be void. The User may not rent, lease, loan, resell, or distribute the Products or any part thereof in any way including, but not limited to, making the Products available to others via shared access to a single computer, a computer network, or by mobile device, digitally or by sharing access information, which includes the User's Username and Password.

3. OWNERSHIP. The Company's Products are the property of the Company, and subject to applicable patent, copyright, trade secrets, trademarks and other proprietary rights. The Products are licensed, not sold, to the User for use only under the terms of this Agreement, and the Company reserves all rights not expressly granted to the User.

4. TERM. This Agreement and license granted herein will terminate at the end of 7 years from the date of purchase.

5. TERMINATION. This Agreement will terminate immediately if the User breaches any term of this Agreement. Further, in the event of a termination or expiration of any agreement between the Company and a third-party content provider or licensor of all or a part of the Products, the User's right to access and use the Products may also terminate or expire without prior notice to User.

6. CONTENT MAINTAINED BY THE COMPANY. User acknowledges and understands that: (a) the Company may, from time to time, elect to update the Products, but the Company does not warrant or guarantee that any Products or other information accessed through the Company's website(s) will be updated at any time during the term of this Agreement; and (b) the Company does not recommend, warrant or guarantee the use or performance of any third-party product or service described in the Products or elsewhere in the Company's website(s), nor is the Company responsible for malfunction of such products or services due to errors in the Products, the User's negligence or otherwise. User agrees to seek additional information on any third-party product or service from the respective third party.

7. WARRANTY DISCLAIMER. EXCEPT AS EXPRESSLY PROVIDED HEREIN, THE COMPANY'S PRODUCTS ARE PROVIDED "AS IS" AND THE COMPANY MAKES NO REPRESENTATIONS OR WARRANTIES. THE COMPANY EXPRESSLY DISCLAIMS ALL WARRANTIES, EXPRESS OR IMPLIED, OF ANY KIND, FOR THE PRODUCTS AND ANY OTHER MATERIAL PROVIDED TO USER BY THE COMPANY, INCLUDING, WITHOUT LIMITATION, THE IMPLIED WARRANTIES OF MERCHANTABILITY, FITNESS FOR A PARTICULAR PURPOSE, AND NON-INFRINGEMENT OF THIRD PARTY RIGHTS. THE COMPANY DOES NOT WARRANT THAT THE PRODUCTS ARE ERROR-FREE, THAT THEIR OPERATION WILL BE UNINTERRUPTED, OR THAT PRODUCTS WILL MEET ANY PARTICULAR USER REQUIREMENTS. WITHOUT LIMITING THE GENERALITY OF THE FOREGOING, THE COMPANY MAKES NO WARRANTY, AND PROVIDES NO ASSURANCE, THAT THE PRODUCTS WILL MEET CERTIFICATION REQUIREMENTS OF ANY REGULATORY AUTHORITY OR OTHER ASSOCIATION LICENSING AGENCY, WITHIN OR OUTSIDE OF THE UNITED STATES.

8. LIMITATION OF LIABILITY. Except as specifically provided herein, neither the Company, its affiliates, agents, authors, or licensors, if any, shall be liable for any claim, demand or action arising out of, or relating to, the User's use of the Products or the Company's performance of (or failure to perform) any obligation under this Agreement or for special, incidental or consequential damages, including, without limitation, damages due to lost revenues or profits, business interruption, or other damages caused by User's inability to use the Products, even if the Company, its affiliates, agents, or licensors have been advised of the possibility of such loss or damages, and whether or not such loss or damages is or are foreseeable.

9. EXPORT LAW. The Company's Products are subject to U.S. export control laws and may be subject to export or import regulations in other countries. Unless in compliance with applicable law and specifically authorized in writing by the Company prior to any Product access, the User shall not export the Products under any circumstances whatsoever. In any case, the User will indemnify and hold the Company harmless from any and all claims, losses, liabilities, damages, fines, penalties, costs and expenses (including reasonable attorneys' fees) arising from, or relating to, any breach by the User of the User's obligations under this section.

10. GOVERNING LAW, JURISDICTION AND VENUE. This Agreement shall for all purposes be governed by and interpreted in accordance with the laws of the State of California as those laws are applied to contracts entered into, and to be performed entirely in California. Any legal suit, action or proceeding arising out of, or relating to this Agreement, shall be commenced in a federal court in California or in state court in California, and each party hereto irrevocably submits to the personal and exclusive jurisdiction and venue of any such court in any such suit, action or proceeding and waives any right which it may have to transfer or change the venue of any such suit, action or proceeding, except that in connection with any suit, action or proceeding commenced in a state court, each party retains the right to remove such suit, action or proceeding to federal court to the extent permissible. The United Nations Convention on Contracts for the International Sale of Goods is specifically excluded from application to this Agreement.

11. ATTORNEY FEES. If any legal action or proceeding is brought for the enforcement of this Agreement or arises from the alleged breach, dispute, default or misrepresentation in connection with any of the provisions of this Agreement, the prevailing party or parties shall be entitled to recover reasonable attorneys' fees and other costs incurred as a result of such legal action or proceeding.

12. WAIVER. No failure to enforce any term of this Agreement shall constitute a waiver of such term in the future unless such waiver so provides by its terms.

13. ASSIGNMENT. Neither this Agreement nor any of the User's rights or obligations hereunder may be assigned by the User in whole or in part without the prior written approval of the Company. Any other attempted assignment shall be null and void.

14. SEVERABILITY. If any part of this Agreement is for any reason found to be invalid, illegal or unenforceable, the validity, legality and enforceability of the remaining provisions of this Agreement shall not be affected and same shall remain in effect.

15. COMPLETE AGREEMENT. This Agreement is the complete and exclusive statement of the agreement between the Company and the User with respect to its subject matter, and supersedes and voids any proposal or prior agreement, oral or written, and any other communications between the parties in relation to its subject matter. No waiver, alteration or modification of this Agreement shall be valid unless made in writing and signed by a corporate officer of the Company.

Table of Contents

APPENDIXES

ACKNOWLEDGMENTS AND CONTRIBUTORS TO THIS ADAPTATION

The team at Kent Intermediate School District, headed by Cheryl Blair, EdD, not only spearheaded the adaptation, but played a critical role in advising, reviewing and piloting adapted activities and materials. The education team included Susan Ekkens, Trude Zbikowski and Erica Becker, Program Facilitators for Kent ISD, and Sara Rumbarger and Steve Taylor, YWCA Facilitators. Special thanks to Renne Wyman, a special education classroom teacher, and Best Prom Ever Director, for her review and pilot of many lessons. Finally, thanks to all the special education teachers and staff who graciously opened their classrooms to this program for Sexual Risk Avoidance Education in Kent, Ionia and Montcalm counties, Michigan.

dfusion's Regina Firpo-Triplett led the adaptation effort with significant contributions by Brittany Lucas, Johanna Kramer and Lizanne Reynolds.

ETR's product development team provided design and copyediting of the adapted curriculum and ancillary materials.

ORIGINAL ACKNOWLEDGMENTS

Making a Difference! An Evidence-Based, Abstinence Approach to Teen Pregnancy, STD and HIV Prevention was developed by Dr. Loretta Sweet Jemmott and Dr. Konstance McCaffree and evaluated by Dr. John Jemmott, III, with the assistance of Dr. Geoffrey T. Fong. These researchers are committed to ensuring that young people have long, healthy and productive lives. They designed and evaluated *Making a Difference!* in the hope of touching the lives of adolescents and reducing their health risks.

Making a Difference! was developed, pilot-tested, implemented and evaluated in a study funded by grant R01 MH52035 from the National Institute of Mental Health. This study was designed to identify the most effective ways to reduce the health risks of middle-school age inner-city youth.

The authors gratefully acknowledge the contributions to this research of Dr. Leonard W. Johnson, Medical Director of the Spruce Medical Center and Director of the Spruce Adolescent, Counseling and Education Program, who facilitated the logistical implementation of the research project; Greer D. Wilson, EdD, Director of Greer & Company, who designed and implemented the facilitator's leadership training component of the study; and Gladys L. Thomas, who coordinated the project.

The authors sincerely appreciate the work of Monique Howard, MPH; Melda Grant, MEd; and Rhonda Wise, BA, who assisted the authors in the preparation of the curriculum for the research project by reviewing curriculum material, typing the curriculum and training the facilitators. The authors acknowledge with deep appreciation the work of Monique Howard, MPH, who created and adapted various activities within the curriculum and tailored them to be appropriate for the population.

The authors would also like to thank Cecelia Cancellaro, Martha Eberhardt, MPH, Lynette Gueits, MHS, and Monique Howard, MPH, who worked diligently and carefully to edit and prepare the curriculum for dissemination. We are also deeply grateful for Monique Howard's and Lynette Gueits's expertise with desktop publishing software that helped prepare the curriculum in a user-friendly format.

Special gratitude is extended to all of the educators, master trainers, facilitators, research assistants, project assistants and clinicians who assisted with or participated in the research on which this curriculum is based.

Finally, a special thank you to all of the young people who participated in the project and whose lives we had the opportunity to touch.

Making a Difference! For Youth with Cognitive Impairments

ABOUT THE DEVELOPERS

Loretta Sweet Jemmott, PhD, RN, FAAN, is a Professor and Director of the Center for Urban Health Research at the University of Pennsylvania's School of Nursing. She is also the co-chair of the Behavior and Social Science Core of Penn's Center for AIDS Research. Dr. Jemmott holds a bachelor's and master's degree in nursing, and a PhD in education, specializing in human sexuality education. For over 25 years, she has designed curricula and implemented various programs for adolescents to reduce STD and pregnancy risk behaviors. Since 1987, she has conducted a series of National Institute of Health–funded randomized controlled trials to develop and evaluate theory-based, developmentally appropriate, behavioral interventions aimed at increasing abstinence and safer sex behaviors among inner-city minority youth in various clinics, schools and community settings. She has published over 56 peer-reviewed articles, books and chapters on this topic. Recognized nationally and internationally as a leader in HIV prevention research with adolescents, she has also been involved in international dissemination activities, including the dissemination, tailoring and training of educators on evidenced-based HIV risk reduction curricula for implementation across the country and around the world, including Jamaica, Mexico, Puerto Rico, Botswana and South Africa. Dr. Jemmott has received numerous prestigious awards for significant contributions to the profession of nursing and education, to the field of HIV prevention research and to the community. Such awards include the Congressional Merit Award and election into the Institute of Medicine, an honor accorded to very few nurses. She is also a Fellow in the American Academy of Nursing. She has served on the National Institute for Nursing Research's Advisory Council, the New Jersey Governor's AIDS Advisory Board, where she co-chaired the Education and Prevention Committee, and the Public Policy Committee for the American Foundation for AIDS Research.

John B. Jemmott, III, PhD, received his PhD in social psychology from the Department of Psychology and Social Relations, Harvard University. After serving as a psychology professor at Princeton University for 18 years, he joined the faculty of the University of Pennsylvania, where he is currently the Kenneth B. Clark Professor of Communication Research in the Annenberg School for Communication and Director of the Center for Health Behavior and Communication in the Annenberg Public Policy Center. Throughout his career, Dr. Jemmott has conducted research on the psychological aspects of physical health. Since 1987, his research has centered on HIV sexual risk reduction among adolescents. Recognized nationally and internationally as a leader in HIV prevention research with adolescents, he has published over 60 articles and book chapters and has received numerous grants from the National Institutes of Health to support his research. Dr. Jemmott has served as a consultant on several research review committees, including the Behavioral Medicine Study

Section, the AIDS and Immunology Research Review Committee and the Office of AIDS Research Advisory Council of the National Institutes of Health. Dr. Jemmott is an elected member of the Academy of Behavioral Medicine Research and the Society of Experimental Social Psychology, and a Fellow of the American Psychological Association and the Society for Behavioral Medicine.

Konstance McCaffree, PhD, CSE, is an associate adjunct professor at Widener University in the Center For Education's Program in Human Sexuality. She is a certified sexuality educator and has been a classroom teacher in the public schools for over 30 years. Dr. McCaffree has taught human sexuality to both elementary and secondary students. Dr. McCaffree served on the Board of Directors of the Sexuality Information and Education Council of the United States (SIECUS) and the Society for the Scientific Study of Sexuality (SSSS) and is active in the American Association of Sexuality Educators Counselors and Therapists (AASECT), serving as the Chair of the Sexuality Education Certification Committee, which establishes standards in sexuality education. Dr. McCaffree conducts workshops nationally and internationally to assist educators and health professionals with their facilitation of sexuality education. In recent years, she has developed curricula and implemented training programs in South Africa, Zambia, Nigeria and the Philippines. She has also been involved with various research projects developing curricula aimed at reducing the risk of HIV/AIDS, sexually transmitted infections, unplanned pregnancy and other health and social problems among teenagers and adults.

Making a Difference! For Youth with Cognitive Impairments

Making a Difference!

For Youth with Cognitive Impairments

FIFTH EDITION

FACILITATOR'S GUIDE

Introduction

In 2018, ETR, dfusion and the Kent Intermediate School District (Kent ISD) in Grand Rapids, Michigan, collaborated to create this adapted version of *Making a Difference!* to serve the special needs of high school students with mild cognitive impairment (MiCI). Kent ISD initiated the adaptation through their Department of Health and Human Services, Administration for Children and Families Grant No: 90SR0003.[1]

Students with MiCI have different instructional needs than their general education peers. Mild cognitive impairment accounts for around 85% of all cognitive disabilities, and students in this category have IQ scores between 55 and 70.[2] Although some students with MiCI can attain reading and math skills at grade levels 3 to 6, some have lower reading levels.[3]

The core content in *Making a Difference!* is appropriate for these students, but the pedagogical approach was adapted to make the information understandable and relevant for students with MiCI.

Adaptation Process

dfusion led the adaptation process with the goal of staying as true as possible to the intentions of the original evidence-based curriculum. All adaptations are considered green- and yellow-light adaptations consistent with the General Adaptation Guidance[4] and red-light adaptations were avoided. The dfusion team worked closely with the multi-disciplinary team at Kent ISD to:

- Delineate the students' learning challenges and the facilitators' implementation challenges during *Making a Difference!* modules, both through conversation and direct observation in the classroom.

- Conceptualize a framework for appropriate adaptations that address the needs of MiCI students and the educators who serve them.

- Create an adapted pilot version of *Making a Difference!* for youth with MiCI, that was piloted in several MiCI classrooms, and refined based on pilot data.

1 This adaptation of the *Making a Difference!* curriculum was made possible by Funding Opportunity Number HHS-2016-ACF-ACYF-SR-1197 from the Department of Health and Human Services, Administration for Children and Families. Its contents are solely the responsibility of Kent Intermediate School District, dfusion and ETR and do not necessarily represent the official views of the Department of Health and Human Services, Administration for Children and Families.

2 Disabled-World.com. (2016). https://www.disabled-world.com/disability/types/cognitive/

3 Healthyplace.com. (2016). https://www.healthyplace.com/neurodevelopmental-disorders/intellectual-disability/mild-moderate-severe-intellectual-disability-differences

4 Firpo-Triplett, R., and Fuller, T. R., (2012). General Adaptation Guidance: A Guide to Adapting Evidence-Based Sexual Health Curricula. ETR and CDC's Division of Reproductive Health.

Adaptation Approach for Students with MiCI

Several learning themes were identified that drove the specific adaptation approaches used. Themes and approaches are outlined below:

Learning Themes	Adaptation Approach
Instruction takes longer, making it difficult to cover all the content in the timeframe. Memory and retention limitations limit building on previously learned information.	• Limit classes to 8–15 students. • Expand the timeframe for modules. • Simplify the number of discussion questions and scenarios, reducing duplication. • Include additional review of previous module learnings at the beginning of each lesson. • Provide parent materials so parents and caregivers can support students' learning of the core concepts and information covered in the modules.
Reading levels are low.	• Eliminate student workbooks and reduce the number of handouts. • Incorporate more graphics.
Many common words need to be defined, in addition to new vocabulary words.	• Simplify new terms in the intervention. • Provide clear definitions as needed for each module. • Provide a glossary of terms for quick reference of simple definitions.
Videos provide too much information to absorb in one sitting.	• Section videos into "chunks" and incorporate pauses to allow the facilitator to check for understanding, reinforce information and highlight important points.
Students struggle to keep on track during small-group work.	• Rework small-group activities as large-group activities, keeping objectives and content aligned with the original activity. • Roleplays are led by the facilitator in the large-group setting.
Students need information on puberty, public/private differences, consent and healthy relationships.	• Incorporate messages about consent and healthy relationships throughout the modules, as they apply. • Add activities in the appendix that cover puberty and the public/private distinction.

Making a Difference! For Youth with Cognitive Impairments

The format of the modules has remained the same, with one exception. Key messages have been called out on the left of the teacher scripts to help facilitators quickly identify key messages embedded in the narrative boxes. Learn more about the pedagogical changes in the Curriculum Teaching Strategies section on page 19.

MiCI Classroom Implementation Guidelines

Implementation guidelines for this version of *Making a Difference!* were created to improve student learning:

- Lead with groups of 15 or fewer youth.

- Lead modules 1 to 3 times per week.

- Lead with classes of youth across multiple years, so the students get reinforcement each year.

- When referring to text in handouts or posters, always read the content aloud and check for understanding.

- If the program is being led by a visiting educator, enlist the assistance of the classroom teacher to:

  » Support the learning of new terms and core concepts between the modules.

  » Distribute the parent letters electronically to each parent.

  » Assist with active activities where the students are moving around the room.

  » Keep the posters up in the classroom or accessible to be used in subsequent modules.

About the Program

Making a Difference! is designed to give young adolescents some of the important tools they need to reduce their risk of pregnancy, HIV and other STDs, and to feel comfortable abstaining from sex. The goal is to increase knowledge and perception of personal vulnerability, develop positive attitudes toward abstinence, and build the refusal/negotiation skills and confidence needed to abstain from sexual intercourse and other sexual behaviors that put them at risk. Abstinence from all behaviors that can cause pregnancy or transmit an STD is the surest way to avoid unplanned pregnancy, HIV and other STDs.

Note: Ideally, young people will receive sexual health education that targets knowledge, attitudes and skills related to both abstinence and safer sex practices such as condom use and contraception. However, for settings in which this approach is not permissible, an evidence-based abstinence-focused program such as **Making a Difference!** *can provide adolescents with support and strategies for choosing abstinence and resisting sexual pressures.*

It isn't easy to motivate people to modify their sexual behavior, even when that behavior puts them at risk. Hence, the model of human behavior used to understand sexual risk behavior in *Making a Difference!* draws upon social learning theories, and the interventions proposed for changing that behavior reflect a cognitive-behavioral approach. The curriculum has also been informed by data gathered through numerous focus groups as well as the developers' extensive experience working with young people.

In order to encourage young people to adopt less risky behaviors they must be provided with the following crucial tools:

- The information they need to understand the issues.

- The cognitive skills that will allow them to examine their beliefs about personal risks and consequences and to analyze the behaviors or situations that increase their risk of pregnancy, HIV and other STDs.

- The intrapersonal (within self) skills to understand and manage their feelings and thoughts.

- The interpersonal (between self and others) skills to define and exercise behaviors that reduce personal risk.

- A sense of self-efficacy or confidence required to allow them to make safer decisions about their sexual choices.

- The motivation to apply these skills to their everyday lives.

The ***Making a Difference!*** curriculum that follows consists of three sections. The first is a Facilitator's Guide that includes information about facilitating the curriculum, the theory behind it and the evaluation of the original curriculum with behavioral findings. It also covers curriculum teaching strategies and format of the intervention modules, including information about group agreements and training strategies, such as brainstorming, roleplaying and interactive activities and games. The second is the ***Making a Difference!*** curriculum itself. The final section, the appendixes, includes optional activities that can be included in the curriculum's implementation, additional information about common STDs, contraceptive methods and drugs, guidelines to managing problem behavior, answers to commonly asked questions and a glossary.

This curriculum is intended to reduce the incidence of vaginal, anal and oral sex among young adolescents and help them make a difference in their lives by making proud and responsible choices about their sexual behavior. The facilitator's ability to deliver the information and conduct the exercises contained in this manual will determine the success of the curriculum, so please take the time to carefully read and understand the basic principles, key elements and content of each session. Our collective efforts can accomplish this goal and have a meaningful impact on the lives of our nation's young people.

Making a Difference! For Youth with Cognitive Impairments

How is "abstinence" reflected or defined in this curriculum?

Making a Difference! is labeled an abstinence-based curriculum because it focuses entirely on knowledge, attitudes and skills that encourage and assist young people in implementing or maintaining abstinence in their relationships. The learning activities, DVDs and scenarios used specifically focus on a clear and direct abstinence message. The additional information and activities provided in the appendixes also support the emphasis on abstinence. In this curriculum, "abstinence" is defined as avoiding vaginal, oral and anal intercourse, as well as any other sexual behaviors that can transmit STDs.

The *Making a Difference!* curriculum does not cover or mention other contraceptive methods or safer sex practices, such as always using latex or polyurethane/polyisoprene condoms, to reduce the risk of unplanned pregnancy, HIV and other STDs. However, youth themselves may ask questions about or otherwise introduce condoms or other birth control methods into the discussion. In contrast to "abstinence-only" curricula, *Making a Difference!* facilitators are encouraged to praise students' questions and statements about effective pregnancy, HIV and other STD prevention methods, even if these include suggestions other than abstinence. Facilitators should NOT denigrate condoms or other effective contraceptive methods, speak of them only in terms of failure rates or exaggerate the rates of failure.

Abstinence is the surest way to avoid unplanned pregnancy, HIV and other STD, and can be a viable choice if adolescents are given accurate information and are allowed to discuss, think about and engage in fun activities that help build the skills needed to practice abstinence successfully. If the comprehensive approach is not an option, young people can still engage in meaningful dialogue and activities around abstinence and their sexual health without demeaning other values and methods.

It is also important to remember that not all adolescent sexual activity is voluntary, and to let young people know that they can choose abstinence at any time, even if they have already had sex. This is particularly important for adolescents who may have been sexually abused.

Overview of the Curriculum

Making a Difference! An Abstinence Approach to Teen Pregnancy, STDs and HIV Prevention is a thirteen-module curriculum designed to empower young adolescents to change their behavior in ways that will reduce their risk of becoming (or getting someone) pregnant, and of becoming infected with HIV or other STDs. Specifically, this curriculum advocates postponing sexual activity and emphasizes that abstinence is the only way to completely eliminate the risk of unplanned pregnancy, HIV and other STDs.

*Note: Ideally, young people will receive sexual health education that targets knowledge, attitudes and skills related to both abstinence and safer sex practices such as condom use and contraception. However, for settings in which this approach is not permissible, an evidence-based abstinence-focused program such as **Making a Difference!** can provide adolescents with support and strategies for choosing abstinence and resisting sexual pressures.*

The original **Making a Difference!** curriculum was designed to be used with smaller groups ranging from six to twelve students, but it can be implemented with larger numbers as well if more time is built into each session. It is appropriate for various community settings, including schools, and youth agencies. This special adaptation of the curriculum for youth with cognitive impairments is divided into thirteen 45- to 60-minute modules and is designed to work in a classroom setting with 15 or fewer students.

Curriculum Objectives

At the completion of the **Making a Difference!** curriculum youth will have:

- Increased knowledge about abstinence as a means of pregnancy, HIV and other STD prevention.
- More positive attitudes/beliefs about abstinence.
- Increased confidence in their ability to negotiate abstinence.
- Increased negotiation skills.
- Stronger intentions to abstain from sex.
- A lower incidence of HIV/STD risk–associated sexual behavior.
- A stronger sense of pride and responsibility in making a difference in their lives.

Making a Difference! For Youth with Cognitive Impairments

Content Outline

The *Making a Difference!* curriculum has four major components. The first component focuses on goals and their relationship to adolescent sexual behavior. The second component emphasizes knowledge, including the causes, transmission and prevention of HIV, other STDs and pregnancy. The third component focuses on beliefs and attitudes about abstinence, pregnancy, STDs and HIV. The fourth stresses skills and self-efficacy including negotiation-refusal skills. It also provides time for practice, reinforcement and support.

Types of Activities

The *Making a Difference!* curriculum includes a series of fun and interactive learning experiences designed to increase participation and help young adolescents understand the risk behaviors that can lead to pregnancy and STDs, including HIV. Activities are designed to help youth feel comfortable practicing abstinence, address their concerns about practicing abstinence and provide strategies for overcoming obstacles to abstinence. For this edition, some activities and teaching strategies have been adapted to better meet the needs of youth with cognitive impairments.

The activities involve viewing DVD clips, playing games, brainstorming, roleplaying, engaging in skill-building exercises and discussions designed to build group cohesion and enhance the learning experience. Each activity is brief, and many require the students to get up out of their chairs and interact with one another. This maintains their interest and attention in a way that lectures or lengthy group discussions do not. Below is a description of the types of activities used, as well as their underlying philosophies and goals.

- The goals activity encourages the adolescents to consider their goals for the future and to think about how participating in sexual activity at their current age might affect the attainment of these goals. It makes clear that the safest strategy for preventing pregnancy, HIV and other STDs is abstaining from sex.

- DVDs are used to depict adolescents in various situations. These DVDs evoke feelings, thoughts, attitudes, beliefs and stereotypes about pregnancy, HIV and other STDs, and the importance of practicing abstinence that are then discussed in a group setting.

- The roleplay scenarios are designed to provide students with the confidence and skills necessary to negotiate abstinence and delay sexual involvement. They also recommend a variety of ways in which the prevention skills learned in this program can be implemented in the students' lives.

- The entire curriculum incorporates the *Making a Difference!* theme designed to encourage the students to be proud of themselves, their families and their communities, and to make a difference in their lives and communities by abstaining from sex.

Training

It is highly recommended that educators who plan to teach *Making a Difference!* receive research-based professional development to prepare them to effectively implement the curriculum with fidelity for the intended target group. ETR provides research-based Training of Educators (TOE) that employs the key components required for quality implementation, including learner engagement, modeling, skills practice and follow-up support. Onsite and regional TOE on *Making a Difference!* is available through ETR's Professional Learning Services. For more information, please visit www.etr.org/ebi/training-ta/types-of-services.

Adapting This Program for Your Population

Program facilitators are encouraged to make minor adaptations (also referred to as "green light" adaptations) to optimize the program for the young people receiving it. Such adaptations are intended to help tailor the curriculum to the needs of participating youth. Examples of minor adaptations include updating statistics and changing the names or editing the language or scenarios in roleplays to better reflect your youth population.

Adaptations such as re-ordering the curriculum lessons or inserting additional content into the middle of the program are considered "yellow light" adaptations because they can have an impact on program flow and effectiveness. It's best to discuss these kinds of changes with the program developers first.

Major changes (also referred to as "red light" adaptations) are discouraged and may significantly affect and alter program effectiveness. Examples of major changes include dropping entire activities or lessons, or altering the key messages of the program.

Adaptation guidelines for evidence-based curricula can be found at www.etr.org/ebi and include additional examples of green-, yellow- and red-light adaptations.

Making a Difference! For Youth with Cognitive Impairments

CURRICULUM COMPONENTS AND FORMAT

Each module included in the *Making a Difference!* curriculum contains different activities. Reduced images of handouts, facilitator materials and posters are included at the end of each module. The first pages of each module explain the following information.

Goals

A set of statements that give the facilitator a reference point for what students will learn from the module.

Learning Objectives

A set of measurable objectives designed to help the facilitator "spot-evaluate" the extent to which a given activity has been successfully completed by the students. Objectives are also listed on the first page of the actitivies designed to meet them.

Strategies/Methods

A list of methods included in the module to achieve the objectives and goals. For example, these may include DVDs, mini-lectures, brainstorming and roleplaying.

Materials Needed

A list of equipment and materials needed for the module and for each specific activity.

Implementation Time / Time Needed

The amount of time allotted to each activity in the module (e.g., Talking Time—10 minutes; Scripted Roleplay—20 minutes). Facilitators should conduct each activity in the time allotted. Facilitators may wish to add time to some of the modules, if possible, to allow for further discussion of DVDs and other activities, or to extend and reinforce the skills practice. A brief activity to review key concepts and clarify new vocabulary is included at the beginning of each module.

Rationale for Each Activity

The rationale for each activity is listed on the first page of the activity. It explains how and why the activity is helpful to students' learning. All materials and exercises contained in the module are designed to help the students to achieve these stated purposes.

Activities

Instructions for implementing each activity are fully described. For example, in the case of a roleplay exercise, the facilitator clearly explains the roles and goals of each character. These exercises are designed to build prevention skills and are an essential part of the program.

Procedures

The procedures for each activity are numbered and include all the steps necessary to implement the activity. Whenever the facilitator is to say a specific instruction or mini-lecture aloud, the material appears in a box.

For example, the procedure would look like this:

1.   **Introduce the activity by saying,**

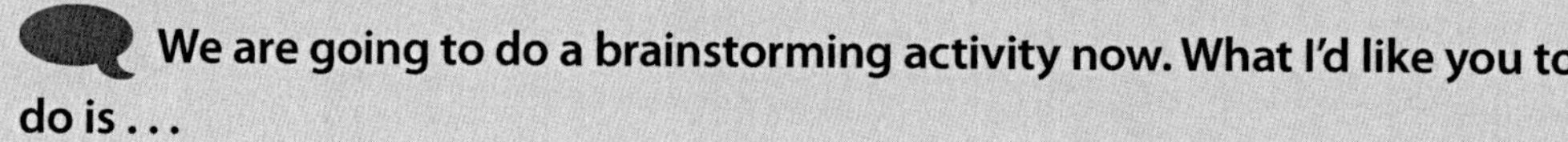

Although it is not necessary to say verbatim what appears in the box, facilitators should be sure that the content and tone are conveyed. Some facilitators find that memorizing the materials works best for them. The group will probably be more attentive if students do not think the facilitator is reading to them.

Key Concepts

For this adaptation of the curriculum, key messages within the facilitator scripts have been called out to the left of the boxes to help facilitators quickly identify the main points to emphasize.

Making a Difference! For Youth with Cognitive Impairments

Facilitator Notes

Facilitator notes give tips to facilitators about implementing the activity. These notes appear at different points in the curriculum where background information or special teaching suggestions are provided. They are contained within a shaded box, as in the following example.

FACILITATOR'S NOTE

Be sure to post the group agreements throughout all the sessions of the program.

Summary Statements

Each activity and module ends with a brief statement from the facilitator about the key take-away messages for students.

THEORETICAL FRAMEWORK

Research shows that curricula are most effective if they are based on a sound theoretical framework. *Making a Difference!* draws upon three theories: the social cognitive theory, the theory of reasoned action, and its extension, the theory of planned behavior. These theories have been shown to be of great value in understanding a wide range of health-related behaviors.

Two major concepts are included in these theories: (1) self-efficacy or perceived behavioral control beliefs, which are defined as people's confidence in their ability to take part in the behavior, e.g., abstain from sex; and (2) outcome expectancies or behavioral beliefs, which are beliefs about the consequences of the behavior. Experience shows that all of the beliefs below are critically important to change behavior. The *Making a Difference!* curriculum addresses each of the principles, usually in more than one activity.

Below is a description of the two types of self-efficacy or perceived behavioral control beliefs emphasized in *Making a Difference!*

Practicing abstinence is easy: "I can do it"

Many young people find it difficult to abstain from sex because of peer pressure, partner pressure and their perception of how others think of them. Therefore, they are less likely to practice abstinence behaviors or negotiate abstinence with their partners. In Module 5, youth examine their attitudes and beliefs about abstinence; in Modules 10 and 11, they learn about peer pressure to have sex; and, in Modules 12 and 13, they learn how to negotiate abstinence with their partners.

Getting your partner to cooperate in practicing abstinence is easy: "I can do it"

Practicing abstinence within a relationship is not something students can do by themselves. They need the cooperation of a partner. Unfortunately, many of students' partners may not be willing. For example, attempts to negotiate abstinence may be interpreted as rejection or lack of physical attraction. Be sensitive to students' desires to maintain their partners' interest and avoid conflict.

At the same time, students need opportunities to practice responding to their partners' objections tactfully and effectively. In Modules 12 and 13, youth are taught negotiation skills that they can practice through roleplays and other interactive exercises.

Below are descriptions of the four types of outcome expectancies or behavioral beliefs emphasized in the *Making a Difference!* curriculum:

Goals Beliefs

The belief that sexual involvement at a young age could have a negative impact on one's goals for the future, including education and a career. In Module 1, the students engage in a Goals activity and discuss obstacles to their goals, including the potentially negative consequences of sex. This belief is incorporated throughout the curriculum.

Prevention Beliefs

The belief that abstinence can eliminate the risk of pregnancy, HIV and other STDs. This belief is incorporated throughout the curriculum.

Partner-Reaction Beliefs

The belief that one's partner would not approve of abstinence and would react negatively to it. This might prevent a person from practicing abstinence. In Modules 10 through 13, students learn how to get out of situations that increase the risk of HIV, other STDs or pregnancy; how to set physical limits; and the negotiation and refusal skills necessary to communicate with their partners about abstinence.

Personal Vulnerability to HIV/STD and Pregnancy Beliefs

Before young people change their behavior they must have a reason or source of motivation to do so. Unless adolescents see how they can personally benefit from doing something differently (for example, practicing abstinence), no amount of skill will be enough to produce change. Many young people do not believe that pregnancy, HIV and other STDs could really happen to them. One goal of *Making a Difference!*, then, is to increase students' sense of personal risk. Personal risk refers to a person's belief that "pregnancy or HIV/STD infection could happen to me." This is addressed throughout the curriculum, but especially in Modules 4, 5, 7, 8 and 9.

UNIQUE FEATURES OF THE CURRICULUM

Making a Difference! has a unique approach that is successful with adolescents. Three major themes serve as the foundation for this curriculum and its implementation.

The Community and Family Approach

A key component of the approach is the strong emphasis on family and community. The importance of protecting one's family and community is used as a motive to change individual behavior. This strategy differs from the traditional approach of HIV prevention, which focused more on protecting oneself as the motive to change risky behavior. The *Making a Difference!* theme encourages adolescents to be proud of themselves and to abstain from sex as a way to prevent sexually transmitted diseases and pregnancy, not only for their own sake, but for the sake of their families and community as well.

This adapted edition includes parent letters with family activities that can be sent home at the end of each module to keep parents/guardians informed about and involved in what students are learning.

The Role of Sexual Responsibility and Accountability

Learning to be sexually responsible and accountable is something that adolescents need to be taught. The *Making a Difference!* curriculum teaches students to make responsible decisions regarding their sexual behavior, urges them to respect themselves and others and stresses the importance of developing a positive self-image. They learn that being responsible and abstaining from sex can contribute to reaching their goals.

The Role of Pride and Making a Difference Through Choosing Abstinence

Adolescence can be a difficult period of development. Adolescents are often faced with confusion, mixed emotions and uncertainty. They are bombarded with sexual messages from various sources, including the media, popular music and their peer group. They are often pressured to be sexually active. They struggle with issues of self-esteem, self-respect and self-pride. Because of this, it is extremely important that they learn to feel good about themselves and their decision to abstain from sex. *Making a Difference!* illustrates that abstaining from sex can actually lead teens to develop a sense of pride, self-confidence and self-respect. The roleplay exercises and other skill-building activities reinforce the many positive benefits, both psychological and physical, of practicing abstinence.

Making a Difference! For Youth with Cognitive Impairments

EVALUATION OF THE ORIGINAL CURRICULUM

Evaluation is a critical component of the *Making a Difference!* program. Many health promotion programs have been implemented in schools, churches, clinics, community-based organizations and other venues, but unfortunately, very few of them include formal evaluation components. Through rigorous research methods, the developers have explored whether or not the interventions designed in this curriculum actually result in the desired outcomes. For example, they set out to determine whether adolescents who participated in the original *Making a Difference!* program did indeed develop more positive outcome expectancies regarding sexual abstinence, and whether such effects were evident up to 12 months after the intervention. Below is a description of the study and its results.

In the research study, the 8-hour curriculum *Making a Difference!* was implemented in a small group setting with African-American male and female adolescents between the ages of 11 and 13 on two consecutive Saturdays in three different middle schools. In this random control trial, 659 6th and 7th grade African-American male and female adolescents, mean age 11.8, were stratified by gender and age and randomly assigned to receive one of three 8-hour curricula: an abstinence curriculum, a safer sex curriculum or a health promotion curriculum (which served as the control group). The adolescents received the curriculum in small groups of six to eight students led by either an African-American adult facilitator (mean age 40) or two peer African American co-facilitators (mean age 16).

The students completed questionnaires before, immediately after and 3, 6, and 12 months after the intervention. Of the original 659 students, 97% returned to complete the 3-month follow-up questionnaire, 94% completed the 6-month, and 93% completed the 12-month follow-up. The primary measures were HIV risk–associated sexual behaviors. The secondary measures were variables from the theory of planned behavior and the social cognitive theory, including knowledge, beliefs, norms, intentions and self-efficacy regarding abstinence.

- The students who received the *Making a Difference!* abstinence curriculum were less likely to report having sexual intercourse in the 3 months after the intervention than were those in the control group.

- *Making a Difference!* delayed sexual experience among students who had not yet had sex. Among the students who reported no previous sexual experience at baseline, the students who received the *Making a Difference!* curriculum were less likely to report having sexual intercourse at the 3-month follow-up than those in the control group.

Other Significant Findings

- The adult and peer facilitators were equally effective. There were no differences in intervention effects on behavior with adult facilitators as compared with peer co-facilitators.

- The adolescents who received the *Making a Difference!* curriculum believed more strongly that practicing abstinence would prevent pregnancy and HIV, expressed less favorable attitudes toward sexual intercourse and reported weaker intentions of having sexual intercourse over the next 3 months than did those in the control group or the safer sex group.

- Adolescents who received *Making a Difference!* also believed more strongly that practicing abstinence would help them achieve their career goals than did those in the control group.

For More In-Depth Information

Jemmott, J. B., III, Jemmott, L. S., and Fong, G. (1998). Abstinence and safer sex HIV risk-reduction interventions for African-American adolescents: A randomized control trial. *Journal of the American Medical Association*, 279 (19): 1529–1536.

Making a Difference! For Youth with Cognitive Impairments

CURRICULUM TEACHING STRATEGIES

Making a Difference! uses several strategies to facilitate behavioral change. Each strategy is defined below and its use in the curriculum is described. Adaptations made to these strategies to better meet the needs of youth with cognitive impairments are identified in the box below each description.

STRATEGY 1: Setting the Environment: The Group Agreements

Module 1 is designed to create a safe, nurturing, non-threatening environment for students, stimulate their interest in the group and provide them with more detailed information about the program. The group agreements that will govern participation in the group should be developed during Module 1. This presentation should permit and encourage discussion designed to give members a sense of participation in the group's decision making. That is, members should be encouraged to accept and live by the standards they agree upon and seek to alter those they wish to change. This is also a good time to provide reassurance to group members about concerns they may have about confidentiality, embarrassment and fear of active participation.

Steps to Creating Group Agreements

- Brainstorm possible agreements.

  For example:
  - » Respect each other's opinions.
  - » One person speaks at a time.
  - » No name-calling.
  - » Confidentiality.
  - » Begin and end on time.

- Clarify and discuss.
- Eliminate any agreements not acceptable to all.
- Come to a group consensus on all agreements.
- Invite students to bring up additions/deletions as the need arises.
- Let students know that everyone is responsible for following and determining the group agreements.

Adaptations for Youth with Cognitive Impairments

- If students have challenges coming up with agreements, make suggestions and ask what they think, or pull ideas from individuals in the group.

- Post the group agreements at the beginning of each session to help students remember them.

General Tips for Improving Group Cohesion and Performance

The following tips can help build group cohesion:

- Frequently reward positive behavior (e.g., during demonstrations or exercises).

- Be supportive.

- Give compliments.

- Be non-judgmental.

- Respect students' feelings and boundaries.

- Model appropriate assertive behavior.

- Be firm when necessary.

- Demonstrate concepts and give examples when possible.

- Keep the language simple.

- Encourage group members to share their experiences at their own pace.

- Build on strengths.

- Listen.

- Let the group members react, think and analyze.

- Be flexible.

- Be patient with the process and try different approaches until you find one that works.

- Clearly convey your expectations for how group members treat each other and how they participate.

- Encourage participation through reinforcement, teaching communication skills, modeling sensitive material, and being supportive, respectful and inclusive regardless of the group members' opinions and beliefs.

- Demonstrate acceptance and respect for all students, regardless of personal characteristics, including race, cultural background, religion, social class, sexual orientation and gender identity.

Making a Difference! For Youth with Cognitive Impairments

STRATEGY 2: Brainstorming

Brainstorming is a technique used to rapidly generate as many ideas as possible, within a given (usually brief) period of time, about a particular question, topic or problem.

For example: Important Concerns of Youth

Students are encouraged to spontaneously express their thoughts and reactions (and the facilitator usually records each idea). No evaluation or criticism of ideas is allowed during this part of brainstorming. Students simply say whatever comes to mind.

For example:

• Family	• School	• Drug use
• Friends	• Relationships	• Getting a job
• Money	• Peer pressure	• Popularity
• Having sex, or not	• Pregnancy	• Music
• Clothes	• Violence	• HIV/AIDS and other STDs

The facilitator may ask probing questions to elicit certain types of ideas or information.

Once a list has been generated, the group then discusses, evaluates and/or processes each idea (giving neither credit nor blame to the person who suggested it).

Adaptations for Youth with Cognitive Impairments

- If students have challenges brainstorming, make suggestions and ask what they think, or pull ideas from individuals in the group.

Positive Characteristics About Brainstorming:

- Permits the facilitator to assess group dynamics: Who are the active members? How does the group respond?
- Builds group cohesion.
- Permits everyone to learn from the information that is generated.
- Permits the opportunity to assess knowledge and skills of the group.

Principles of Brainstorming:

- Try to get out as many ideas as possible.

- Students can say anything that comes to mind.

- DON'T EVALUATE IDEAS; a later time can be set aside for evaluation.

- DON'T DISCUSS SUGGESTIONS; a later time can be set aside for discussion.

- Allow repetition.

- Encourage everyone's participation.

- Encourage building on other ideas.

- Allow periods of silence.

STRATEGY 3: Interactive Activities and Competitive Games

Interactive activities and competitive games give the students the opportunity to practice what they learned. One of the best strategies for teaching young people is to use fun, interactive and competitive activities, and many such activities are included in this curriculum.

Games and activities are a good strategy for teaching content. Games often promote rich discussion as students work hard to prove their points. Because games can promote competition, remind students of the group agreements prior to the game.

Facilitators—remember to read the instructions and game rules prior to teaching the game, and make adaptations as necessary.

STRATEGY 4: Processing a DVD or Game

The practice of processing after an activity allows students to reflect upon what they learned/experienced. Processing also allows the facilitator to draw out the key points of the activity. The most common way to process is to ask a series of questions or make a series of statements.

For example:

- Ask questions designed to elicit discussion.

  General Reactions

  » What did you think of the DVD?

Making a Difference! For Youth with Cognitive Impairments

» What is your response to the activity?

» How do you think Pat felt when…?

- Encourage all students to contribute. In some groups, there are a few students who may be less willing to volunteer during the discussion. The following techniques may be used to encourage all students to contribute.

Personal Reactions

» How did you feel about…?

» Describe what you saw.

» What will you do as a result of…?

Adaptations for Youth with Cognitive Impairments

- Because videos may provide too much information for students to absorb in one sitting, section videos into "chunks." Places to pause the DVD are identified in the procedures.

- During the pauses, facilitators can check for understanding, reinforce information and highlight important points.

STRATEGY 5: Working in Small Groups

Adaptations for Youth with Cognitive Impairments

- Because students may struggle to keep on track with small-group work, these activities from the original *Making a Difference!* curriculum have been reworked as large-group activities and discussions.

- For example, the facilitator reads scenarios aloud and discusses with the full group, recording main points on newsprint or the board.

- Objectives and content remain aligned with the original activities, but working with the full group allows facilitators to monitor and assist all students as needed.

STRATEGY 6: Roleplaying / Practice

This method of acting out imaginary situations allows students to practice using a new skill. It provides an opportunity for students to take risks with new ways of behaving in a safe situation without fear of failure, and to see how their peers will react to their behavior.

Adaptations for Youth with Cognitive Impairments

- Roleplays are led by the facilitator in the large-group setting.

- Facilitators can prepare chart paper ahead of time with the lines written out and blank spaces for the responses students will generate as a group.

- Facilitators can choose strong readers for the scripted roleplays, or play one or both of the roles themselves, if needed.

- For unscripted roleplays, facilitators take on the role of the person pressuring and work with a student volunteer to present the roleplay.

- If students seem ready, facilitators may choose to have two students perform together. Assign each student a role (i.e., person being pressured and person pressuring) and be sure to explain their goals in the roleplay before it begins.

- Non-roleplaying students act as observers and give feedback on the roleplay.

Tips for Making Roleplays Successful

- Set and follow norms or ground rules for group behavior.

- See yourself as the director of a movie.

- Make every effort to allow students to volunteer. Urge everyone to participate.

- Set the scene.

- Rehearse.

- Record to ensure transfer.

- Start with low-risk situations and move to high-risk situations. It may be beneficial to begin with scripted roleplays and then move to unscripted roleplays.

- Give continuous positive reinforcement.

 Making a Difference! For Youth with Cognitive Impairments

GENERAL TIPS FOR PREPARING TO IMPLEMENT THE CURRICULUM

- Review the curriculum manual ahead of time.

- Review the format of the manual, which consists of goals, objectives, preparation, materials and a detailed outline of what the facilitator should say and do for each activity.

- Become familiar with all activities, DVDs and curriculum materials.

- Make sure you have all the necessary equipment and materials.

- Review the supplemental background information provided in Appendix B about HIV, other STDs, contraceptive methods and effects of alcohol and other drugs.

- Learn about local resources such as health departments and family planning clinics.

- Know the policies of school districts and community agencies in regard to implementing new programs, discussing issues of sexuality and gaining parental support and permission.

Materials

Making a Difference! uses the following materials at various points in the curriculum. Use this checklist to prepare for teaching. Some of the items will need to be prepared prior to beginning the sessions; others can be developed as part of the process.

Materials Needed (Not Included in Implementation Kit)

Masking tape

Markers

Pencils/pens (enough for each student)

Newsprint

Monitor and device for showing DVDs

Index cards (2 labeled D, 6–7 labeled A, the remainder labeled U)

Blank index cards

Bag or box large enough to hold several items (optional)

Various puberty-related hygiene and personal care products (optional)

Pre-Labeled Newsprint

Group Agreements

Making a Difference! Be Proud! Be Responsible!

Goals (written on left side of newsprint)

Why Some Young People Have Sex

Consequences of Sex

Proud and Responsible Prevention Strategies

Benefits of Sex/Abstinence

How STDs Are Transmitted

Reasons to Avoid STDs

Benefits of Waiting

Delaying Strategies

Characteristics of Healthy Relationships (optional)

Characteristics of Unhealthy Relationships (optional)

Materials Included in Implementation Kit

Cards

Risk Behavior cards

Public or Private Bingo cards (optional)

Posters

Body Changes

Female Body — Outside

Female Body — Inside

Male Body — Inside

How Do People Express Their Sexual Feelings?

HIV/AIDS Review

Key Words

Risk Continuum signs

Agree/Disagree signs

STOP, THINK and ACT

STD

Signs of STDs

Showing Physical Affection signs

Consent

Making a Difference! For Youth with Cognitive Impairments

Refuse

How to Say "NO"

Examples of a Strong "NO"

Explain Why

Suggest Other Activities

Roleplay Guidelines

Public or Private Places (optional)

TREO (optional)

Handouts

Goals Timeline

Seeing the Positive

Calling Koko Callers (1–3)

Your Birthday Gift (Scripted Roleplay)

Jamal and Keisha

Peer Pressure Scenarios 1–4

While They're Out (Scripted Roleplay)

While They're Out (Unscripted Roleplay)

DVDs

The Subject Is Puberty (Abstinence Version)

The Subject Is HIV (Abstinence Version)

Tanisha & Shay

Background Reading

Jemmott, J. B., III, Fry, D., and Jemmott, L. S. (2009). Abstinence interventions. In A. O'Leary (Ed.), *Beyond Condoms*. New York: Plenum.

Jemmott, J. B., III, and Jemmott, L. S. (2008). Helping adolescents reduce their risk of AIDS. In M. Chesney (Ed.), *Health Psychology and HIV Disease*. New York: Plenum.

Jemmott, J. B., III, and Jemmott, L. S. (2001). HIV risk-reduction behavioral interventions with heterosexual adolescents. *AIDS*, 14 (suppl 2): S40–S52.

Jemmott, J.B. III, and Jemmott, L. S. (2000). HIV behavioral interventions for adolescents in community settings. In J. L. Peterson and R. J. DiClemente (Eds.), *Handbook of HIV Prevention*. New York: Plenum.

Jemmott, L. S. (2000). Saving our children: Strategies to empower African-American adolescents to reduce their risk for HIV infection. *Journal of National Black Nurses Association*, 2 (1): 4–14.

Jemmott, J. B., III, and Jemmott, L. S. (1999). Reducing HIV risk-associated sexual behaviors among African American adolescents: Testing the generalizability of intervention effects. *Journal of Community Psychology*, 27: 161–187.

Jemmott, J. B., III, Jemmott, L. S., and Fong, G. (1998). Abstinence and safer sex HIV risk-reduction interventions for African-American adolescents: A randomized control trial. *Journal of American Medical Association*, 279: 1529–1536.

Jemmott, J. B., III, and Jemmott, L. S. (1994). Interventions for adolescents in community settings. In R. DiClimente and J. Peterson (Eds.) *Preventing AIDS : Theory and Practice of Behavioral Interventions*. New York: Plenum.

Jemmott, J. B., III, Jemmott, L. S., and Hacker, C. (1992). Predicting intentions to use condoms among African American adolescents: The theory of planned behavior as a model of HIV risk associated behavior. *Journal of Ethnicity and Disease*, 2: 371–380.

Jemmott, J. B., III, Jemmott, L. S., Spears, H., Hewitt, N., and Cruz-Collins, M. (1992). Self-efficacy, hedonistic expectancies, and condom-use intentions among inner-city black adolescent women: A social cognitive approach to AIDS risk behavior. *Journal of Adolescent Health*, 13: 512–519.

Jemmott, J. B., III, Jemmott, L. S., and Fong, G. (1992). Reductions in HIV risk-associated sexual behaviors among black male adolescents: Effects of an AIDS prevention intervention. *American Journal of Public Health*, 82: 372–377.

Making a Difference! For Youth with Cognitive Impairments

Making a Difference!

For Youth with Cognitive Impairments

FIFTH EDITION

CURRICULUM

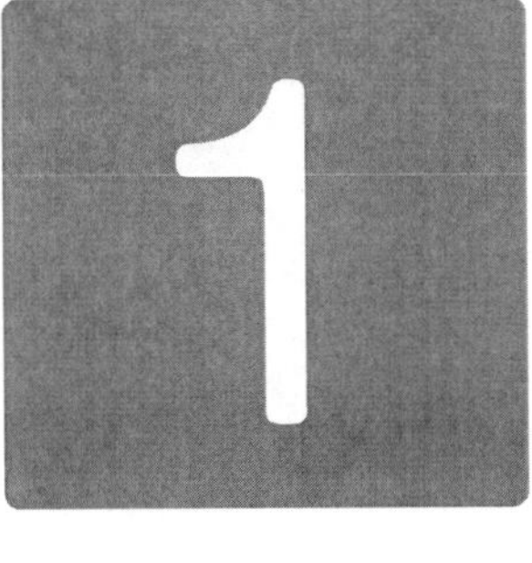

GETTING TO KNOW YOU AND STEPS TO MAKING YOUR GOALS COME TRUE

GOALS

The goals of this module are to:

- Provide students with an overview of the program.

- Increase students' personal investment and comfort in participating in the program.

- Increase students' ability to identify realistic goals for their future.

- Increase students' confidence about making proud and responsible choices to protect themselves and their community from unplanned pregnancy, HIV and other STDs.

LEARNING OBJECTIVES

After completing this module, students will be able to:

- Identify several agreements for group participation that will facilitate discussion and learning.

- Identify what it means to be proud and responsible.

- Describe the benefits of proud and responsible behavior.

- Describe at least one goal they wish to achieve in the future.

- Identify barriers to achieving their personal goals and strategies for overcoming them.

MODULE PREVIEW

The first module: (1) informs students about the program; (2) helps them become comfortable, cohesive and productive in groups; (3) generates enthusiasm about *Making a Difference!* (4) promotes the goal of protecting themselves and their community; and (5) gives them ideas about how they can examine their own goals, and obstacles that might stand in the way of reaching them.

STRATEGIES/METHODS

- Mini-Lecture
- Brainstorming
- Talking Time Exercise
- Goals and Obstacles Exercise
- Group Discussion

MATERIALS NEEDED — INCLUDED IN IMPLEMENTATION KIT

Goals Timeline handout

MATERIALS NEEDED — NOT INCLUDED IN IMPLEMENTATION KIT

- Pencils/pens
- Markers
- Masking tape
- Pre-labeled newsprint:
  - » *Group Agreements*
  - » *Making a Difference! Be Proud! Be Responsible!*
  - » *Goals and Obstacles*

PREPARATION NEEDED

1. Label all of the newsprint charts as listed under Materials.

2. Hang the pre-labeled newsprint charts in the order they will be used. Fold and tape the charts so the titles remain covered by the bottom half of the sheet until you use them.

3. Prepare to review and define the following terms (definitions in the glossary) throughout the lesson as needed:

   - » abstinence
   - » behavior
   - » future
   - » goal
   - » I-statement
   - » obstacle
   - » pregnancy
   - » proud
   - » respect
   - » responsible
   - » sex
   - » sexuality
   - » sexually transmitted disease (STD)
   - » transgender
   - » transmitted
   - » value

INSTRUCTIONAL TIME: 45–60 minutes

ACTIVITY	MINUTES NEEDED
Pre-Activity: Introduce Key Terms	5
A. **Welcome and Program Overview**	5
B. **Talking Time**	10–12
C. **Creating Group Agreements**	5–8
D. ***Making a Difference! Be Proud! Be Responsible!* Brainstorm**	5–8
E. **Goals Timeline**	10–15
F. **Brainstorming Obstacles to Your Goals**	5–7

 Making a Difference! For Youth with Cognitive Impairments

PREPARING FOR THE ACTIVITY

RATIONALE

Providing students with a brief overview of key terms to be used in the module will prime them for new learning.

MATERIALS

None

TIME

5 minutes

PROCEDURE

1. Define any terms from this module that you expect your students will need to have defined before beginning the lesson. Terms may include:

» abstinence	» obstacle	» sex	» transgender
» behavior	» pregnancy	» sexuality	» transmitted
» future	» proud	» sexually transmitted disease (STD)	» value
» goal	» respect		
» I-statement	» responsible		

PREPARING FOR THE ACTIVITY

RATIONALE

Providing students with a general overview of the program will foster excitement and enthusiasm about participating.

MATERIALS

None

TIME

5 minutes

PROCEDURE

1.   Welcome the students and introduce yourself.

2.   Present the purpose and format of the program by saying,

KEY MESSAGE:

This program is about helping you avoid unplanned pregnancy and diseases that are transmitted through having sex.

Some teens don't know about STDs. Some teens don't know how babies are made or how hard it is to be a parent. This program will teach about STDs and pregnancy and how to avoid them.

This program is called *Making a Difference!* It will give you some important tools to protect yourself and others from unplanned pregnancy and sexually transmitted diseases—STDs.

This program teaches information and skills for you to avoid pregnancy and STDs. It also teaches about relationships, sexual behavior, decision making and dealing with difficult situations. Learning this information will help you to protect yourself from getting pregnant or becoming infected with STDs.

(continued)

KEY MESSAGE:

If people have sex without
protection, they could create
a pregnancy or get a disease.

Sexual activity may interfere
with your goals.

> *(continued)*
>
> Although STDs can be avoided, many young people
> don't take steps to protect themselves because
> they don't believe they are at risk of getting an STD.
> Anyone can get an STD from having unprotected sex
> with a partner who is infected.
>
> Unplanned pregnancies can be avoided too. Many
> teen parents make successful lives for themselves and
> their children, but it's a lot of hard work. It's easier to
> reach your goals if you wait to have a child.

3. Ask students if they think young people should be worried about unplanned
   pregnancy and STDs. Allow students to answer.

4a. Tell students that the people who wrote this program care about the lives of young
    people, and want them to have the information and skills to protect themselves from
    unplanned pregnancy and STDs.

4b. Then say,

KEY MESSAGE:

This program has lots of fun
activities and games that
will help you learn to protect
yourself and others from
unplanned pregnancy and
STDs.

> To make the program interesting and fun, it includes
> DVDs, exercises and games that I hope you will enjoy.
> Although the information is serious and important, I
> hope we can learn together and have a good time.

5. Ask if anyone has questions. Answer any questions students have about the purpose
   or format of the program.

6. Tell students that now that they have an idea of what to expect, it's time to get started.

FACILITATOR'S NOTE

STD or STI? Some health educators prefer the term "STI" (sexually transmitted infection) over "STD" (sexually transmitted disease), whereas others use the two interchangeably. This intervention, along with the Centers for Disease Control and Prevention and many other leaders in health education, uses STD because this is the term understood by the greatest number of people, including teens. It is important for everyone to understand that STDs (STIs) can present with or without symptoms.

PREPARING FOR THE ACTIVITY

RATIONALE

Opening and closing each day with Talking Time encourages students to feel like important contributors to the group and gives them an opportunity to express their thoughts and feelings.

MATERIALS

None

TIME

10–12 minutes

PROCEDURE

1a. Explain Talking Time,

KEY MESSAGE:

Talking Time allows us to get to know one another by sharing a little bit about ourselves.

Talking Time is a communication tool used to bring people together to teach, learn, listen and share.

We will use Talking Time each class to check-in and get to know a little about each other.

1b. Tell the group you will go around the room so each person will have a chance to speak. Let students know that they may pass if they are not ready when it is their turn, and the group will come back to them at the end.

1c. Explain what to share during Talking Time,

KEY MESSAGE:

Share your name, age, and something else about yourself you want us to know.

Let's try Talking Time by using it to introduce ourselves. I will speak first and when it is your turn please share your name, your age and something else you'd like us to know about you, like a hobby or favorite activity.

2. Model the Talking Time process by beginning with yourself,

My name is _____________________ and I am _____________________ (age).

I like to… *(share something you enjoy doing)*.

FACILITATOR'S NOTE

If helpful for the students, post "Name, Age, Something About Me" on the board for reference.

3. Ask for a volunteer to start. Encourage each student to speak. When Talking Time is complete, thank each person for sharing.

4. Summarize this activity,

KEY MESSAGE:

Sharing and learning about each other is important. During this program we'll get to know one another better and learn what's important to each of us.

Thanks to all of you for sharing a little about yourselves. During the program, we will get to know more about each other and what is important to each of us. Talking Time is now over, but we will use it again later.

 Making a Difference! For Youth with Cognitive Impairments

FACILITATOR'S NOTE

You can also use alternative sentence stems in the introductions. Here are some ideas:

* One of my favorite TV shows or movies is _______________________.

* The best movie I've ever seen is _______________________.

* The best book I've ever read is _______________________.

PREPARING FOR THE ACTIVITY

RATIONALE

Group agreements increase trust among students and help facilitators provide structure when discussions become difficult or awkward. Developing guidelines as a group builds cohesion and increases the likelihood that the agreements will be followed.

ACTIVITY LEARNING OBJECTIVE

- Identify agreements for group participation that will facilitate discussion and learning.

MATERIALS

- Pre-labeled newsprint (example right):
  - » *Group Agreements*
- Markers
- Masking tape

TIME

5–8 minutes

Group Agreements

PROCEDURE

1. Begin this activity by unfolding the pre-labeled newsprint titled *Group Agreements* and saying,

KEY MESSAGE:

Group agreements are guidelines that will help us feel safe and comfortable to talk about sensitive topics like sex in this program.

> We're going to be talking about sexuality—a topic that sometimes can cause people to feel nervous or uncomfortable. What guidelines or agreements could we put in place to help make sure that everyone in the group feels safe, comfortable and able to participate?

2. Have students brainstorm a list of agreements or guidelines for the group to follow. As the students offer guidelines, write them on the newsprint titled *Group Agreements*.

FACILITATOR'S NOTE

If students have challenges brainstorming, pull ideas from individuals in the group.

3. Make sure the list includes confidentiality, right to pass and respecting diversity. You may also include some of the other following suggestions.

KEY MESSAGE:

Agreements should include "Confidentiality." This means that everyone keeps what is said here in this group private.

No one should share any personal information we hear in this group.

The one exception to this is if any of you tell me something that might cause you or someone else harm, I will have to tell someone for safety reasons—for example, if you told me you were going to hurt yourself or someone else, or if someone talks about being abused in any way.

GROUP AGREEMENTS AND GUIDELINE SUGGESTIONS

Confidentiality: When people share private information in this group, it should be kept private. If, for example, someone shares about crying because of hurt feelings, do not discuss or joke about this with someone outside the group. We will not talk about any personal information we hear in this group with people outside this group.

There is one exception. If any of you tell me something that might cause you or someone else harm, I will have to tell someone for safety reasons— for example, if you told me you were going to hurt yourself or someone else, or if someone talks about being abused in any way. Please know that it is important to tell and to get help if you or someone else is being harmed. You can talk to me or another trusted adult outside of this group.

No put-downs: Show respect for others, even if you disagree with them. If someone says something that you disagree with, do not say, "that's stupid" or "you're wrong." You can say you have a different idea and share it. All questions are important. There is no such thing as a "silly question."

(continued)

KEY MESSAGE:

Agreements should include "Right to Pass." This means you don't have to share unless you want to.

KEY MESSAGE:

Let me know if anything makes you feel uncomfortable during our sessions.

(continued)

GROUP AGREEMENTS AND GUIDELINE SUGGESTIONS

Be supportive of each other: We will be discussing important and sometimes personal information about making choices and risky behaviors. At times you may talk about yourself, your peers and your partners. It is important that we respect each other by not laughing at anyone or making statements that put people down.

Use "I-statements": In this group, it is important to talk about how YOU feel, think or act and not about how you think "all teens" or "all your friends" feel, think or act.

Right to pass: Sometimes when talking about subjects like sex, someone might not want to talk or might have an uncomfortable feeling or memory. If you ever feel like being quiet or not sharing, it's OK to just listen. If I call on you or someone asks you a question, you can say, "I pass." All group members are allowed to not answer any question they do not want to.

Step up, step back: If you usually talk a lot, step back sometimes so others can talk. If you are usually quiet, step up and participate a little more so the group can benefit from your ideas.

Dealing with discomfort: Sometimes topics can bring up uncomfortable feelings for people. If anything makes you feel uncomfortable during our sessions, let me know. If you need to step outside for a few minutes, we can arrange that. Please come to me with any concerns you have. If I can't help, I can connect you with people that can.

KEY MESSAGE:

Agreements should include "Respect Diversity." This means we understand that people are different and treat everyone with respect.

KEY MESSAGE:

Regardless of our differences, everyone is welcome in this group. It is a safe space for everyone.

Respect diversity: Let's remember that there's diversity in this group. People come from different family backgrounds, racial and cultural groups, and living situations. Some young people have already had romantic relationships; others aren't even thinking about it. Some may have had sexual intercourse. Some may have had sex because they chose to; others may have had sex against their will. Some people are interested in romantic relationships with people of the same sex; others are interested in the opposite sex. Some may identify as male, female or transgender. All of these differences make us unique. Regardless of how you see yourself, your background, previous relationships or experience, each of you has a place in this group. This will be a safe space for everyone.

Other agreements you should include if students do not mention them:

- Listen to others.

- Don't interrupt.

- Allow everyone to participate.

4. Ask students if they have any other suggestions they would like to add.

5. Once the list is complete, re-read each agreement and ask all students to nod and say "yes" that they agree to follow that guideline.

6. Summarize this activity by saying,

KEY MESSAGE:

Our group agreements will be posted every time we meet to help us remember them.

You did a great job creating the list! I will post our group agreements each time we meet so we can all see it and remember those guidelines.

I am excited and feel that we can work well together and respect each other by following our group agreements. I look forward to working with all of you.

If the class already has group agreements in place, ask students to share them. If not already included, add agreements about confidentiality, right to pass, and respecting diversity.

Be sure to post the group agreements throughout all the sessions of the program.

Making a Difference! For Youth with Cognitive Impairments

MAKING A DIFFERENCE! BE PROUD! BE RESPONSIBLE! BRAINSTORM

PREPARING FOR THE ACTIVITY

RATIONALE

This activity introduces the theme of the program, *"Making A Difference! Be Proud! Be Responsible!"* The emphasis on being proud and responsible provides a motivation for engaging in health-protective behavior and for encouraging others to do the same.

ACTIVITY LEARNING OBJECTIVES

- Identify what it means to be proud and responsible.
- Describe the benefits of proud and responsible behavior.

MATERIALS

- Pre-labeled newsprint (example right):
  - » *Making a Difference! Be Proud! Be Responsible!*

TIME

5–8 minutes

> *Making a Difference!*
>
> *Be Proud!*
>
> *Be Responsible!*

PROCEDURE

1. Tape the *Making a Difference! Be Proud! Be Responsible!* newsprint on the wall.

2. Open the discussion by introducing the title of the program, *Making a Difference!*

3a. Explain that as a group students are going to do some brainstorming, where everyone just says whatever comes to mind about a particular issue or question.

3b. Tell students they are going to brainstorm the answers to three questions:

   (1) What does it mean to make a difference?

   (2) What does it mean to be proud?

   (3) What does it mean to be responsible?

4. Have students brainstorm answers to these questions. Record their answers on the newsprint.

    » **Making a Difference** means taking action and making positive changes. It means doing things that you feel good about, that your family and community will respect and that will help you achieve your goals.

    » To **Be Proud** is to feel happy and pleased about something you've done or accomplished, to feel that you have lived up to your expectations or behaved according to your own or community values.

    » To **Be Responsible** is to be dependable, dedicated, reliable, committed, truthful and trustworthy.

5a. Explain what *pride* and *responsibility* mean,

KEY MESSAGE:

You are all worthy people who have value. Being proud and responsible means knowing that and showing it with your choices.

Being proud and responsible means that you value yourself and you believe you are worthy! Each one of you has value. Each one of you is worthy. You have to behave in ways that show you understand your worth.

 Making a Difference! For Youth with Cognitive Impairments

5b. Explain what being *abstinent* means,

KEY MESSAGE:

The surest way to protect yourself from unplanned pregnancy and STDs is choosing to be abstinent, or not do any sexual behaviors that could cause pregnancy or spread disease. This is a proud and responsible choice.

Proud and responsible behavior also can apply to sex. It means you understand that the surest way to protect yourself from unplanned pregnancy and STDs is to be *abstinent,* which means choosing not to do any sexual behaviors that could cause pregnancy or spread diseases.

5c. Bring up issues related to sexual abuse,

KEY MESSAGE:

Sometimes people are forced to do sexual behaviors they don't want to. If you are in a situation where you aren't able to make your own choices about sexual activity, please tell me or another trusted adult to get help.

We know that some young people have been sexually abused, and they didn't get to make a choice about doing sexual behaviors. Youth who have survived something like that can use that inner strength in the future and choose to wait to have sex in order to protect themselves from STDs and unplanned pregnancies. If you are currently in a situation where you don't get to make your own choices about sexual activity, please reach out to me or another trusted adult to get help.

6. Then ask what students think are some benefits of practicing proud and responsible behaviors.

Make sure answers include:

- » Feel better about yourself.
- » Have healthier relationships.
- » Stay out of trouble.
- » Accomplish your goals.
- » Make people feel proud of you.
- » Reduce your risk of pregnancy, HIV and other STDs.
- » Have a healthier body.
- » Stay in school.
- » Feel like you are helping your loved ones and your community.

7. Conclude,

KEY MESSAGE:

A proud and responsible thing you can do is to choose to be abstinent from sexual behaviors to avoid unplanned pregnancy and STDs.

I believe that you can make a difference, and feel proud and responsible. One proud and responsible thing young people can do is to abstain from any sexual behavior that could cause pregnancy or diseases. People who engage in responsible behavior can feel proud because they help protect themselves and their friends, families and communities.

Making a Difference! For Youth with Cognitive Impairments

PREPARING FOR THE ACTIVITY

RATIONALE

To achieve their goals, students need to think about their future and to understand that their present behavior will have an impact on what they will be doing 5 and 10 years from now.

ACTIVITY LEARNING OBJECTIVE

- Describe at least one goal for the future.

MATERIALS

- Pencils
- *Goals Timeline* handout
- Pre-labeled newsprint (example right):
  - » *Goals and Obstacles* (Write "Goals" on the left side of newsprint, and leave room for "Obstacles" on the right side)

<table>
<tr><td>**Goals**</td><td></td></tr>
<tr><td></td><td></td></tr>
</table>

TIME

10–15 minutes

PROCEDURE

1. Introduce the exercise by explaining that the next activity will help students take a look at their past, present and future.

FACILITATOR'S NOTE

Record some events from your own life on a copy of the *Goals Timeline* handout. Provide examples for each section. This will help students understand what you want them to do.

2a. Distribute the *Goals Timeline* handout. Explain that this timeline will help students think about what they have already accomplished and what they want to accomplish someday.

2b. In the first section, have students think about and write down something they have done that made them really proud. Give examples: playing for a sports team, getting certain grades, attending a particular social event, joining a club, winning a student election, artistic or musical performance, etc. Give students a few minutes to complete the first task.

3. Move on to the second section of the timeline. Instruct students to imagine themselves 1 year out of high school. Have them think of and write down at least one goal, something they hope to achieve by then that will make them proud. Give students a few minutes to complete the second task.

4. Ask volunteers to share their goals from the second section, and record answers on the newsprint under the "Goals" section.

5. Now, have students imagine that they're adults who are 25 years old. Ask them to think of and write down at least one thing they hope to achieve by that age that will make them proud. Allow a few minutes for students to complete their timelines.

6. Again, ask students to share, and record answers on the newsprint under the "Goals" section.

7. Compliment students' hard work and the goals they identified.

8.   Now, have students think about just one of their goals. Ask what they need to do for it to happen.

9.   Give students a few minutes to share their ideas and strategies.

10. Compliment students on their answers.

11. Summarize the activity by saying,

KEY MESSAGE:

Making proud and responsible choices will help you to reach your goals.

You can reach your goals with a little planning and organizing, and by making proud and responsible decisions. Reaching your goals will make you and the people you care about proud. Remember that you are capable of doing whatever you put your mind to.

BRAINSTORMING OBSTACLES TO YOUR GOALS

PREPARING FOR THE ACTIVITY

RATIONALE

Directing students' attention to the potential obstacles they may face when pursuing their goals encourages them to develop strategies to avoid, surmount or reduce those obstacles.

ACTIVITY LEARNING OBJECTIVE

- Identify barriers to achieving goals and strategies for overcoming them.

MATERIALS

- Pre-labeled newsprint (example right):
  » *Goals and Obstacles* (from the previous activity)
- Markers
- Masking tape

Goals	Obstacles

TIME

5–7 minutes

PROCEDURE

1. Refer to the *Goals and Obstacles* newsprint from the previous activity.

2. Write "Obstacles" on the right side of the newsprint.

3. Explain to students that now that they've listed their goals, you're going to talk about obstacles, things that might prevent them from achieving those goals. Ask them to brainstorm obstacles that may get in the way of their goals.

   Answers should include:

   » Unplanned pregnancy, HIV and other STDs

4. Write their responses under "Obstacles" on the right side of the *Goals and Obstacles* newsprint with a different colored marker.

5. Say,

KEY MESSAGE:

Obstacles can change your life and make it harder to achieve your goals.

> If you've already encountered any of these obstacles, you understand how your life can change. Things can work out just fine but it can be a lot harder to reach your goals.

6a. Ask how the obstacles listed can be avoided, and elicit some responses.

6b. Ask what people can do to make sure they don't get pregnant, get someone pregnant, or get an STD, such as HIV, and elicit some responses.

7. Pick a few of the key obstacles and discuss ways to avoid, overcome or reduce them. If there are any teen parents in the group, ask them to discuss ways they have been able to manage the additional responsibility of raising a child and still accomplish their goals.

8. Summarize by saying,

KEY MESSAGE:

Being abstinent is a proud and responsible choice that will help you reach your goals.

> I'm impressed with your goals. For the rest of the program we will be looking at ways to overcome obstacles so that you can reach your goals. Being abstinent is a choice that can protect you and help you reach your goals despite obstacles.

KEY MESSAGE:

You are all worthy of getting the good things you want for your future.

> You're worthy of all the good things you imagine for your future. Each time we meet you'll gain knowledge, beliefs and skills to empower you to make a difference! I look forward to working with you.

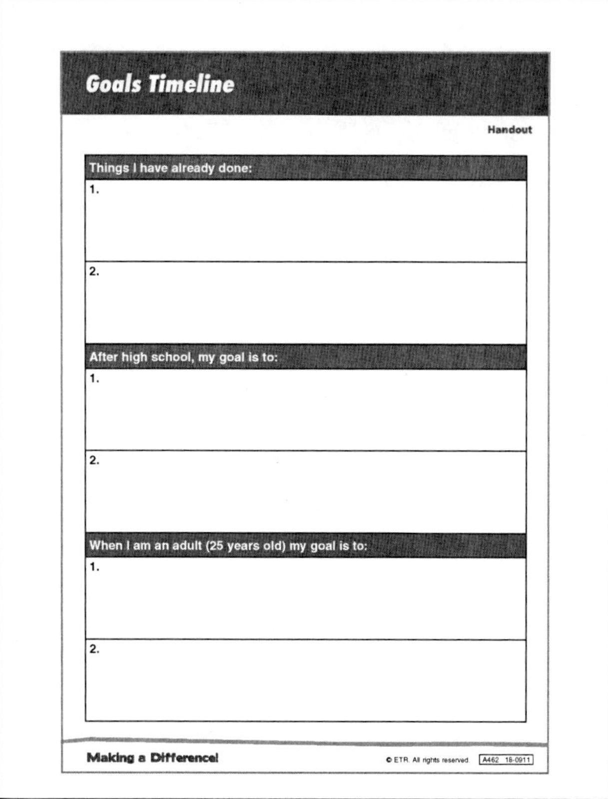

Handout

Making a Difference! For Youth with Cognitive Impairments

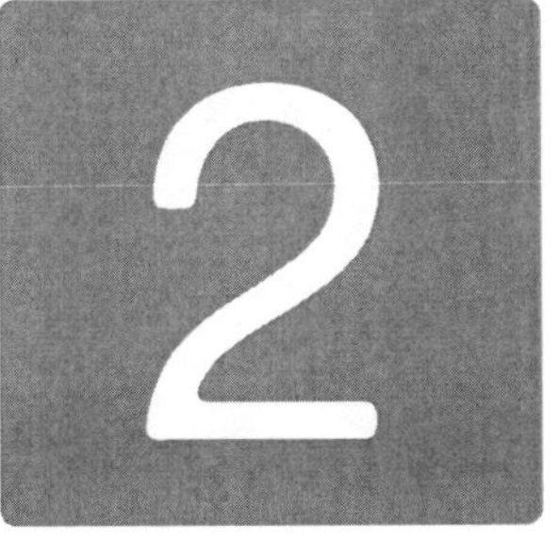

MODULE 2

UNDERSTANDING ADOLESCENT SEXUALITY

GOALS

The goals of this module are to:

- Review information about why young people have sex.
- Increase students' knowledge about physical, emotional and sexual development associated with puberty.
- Increase students' awareness of the pressures to become involved in sexual activity.

LEARNING OBJECTIVES

After completing this module, students will be able to:

- Identify the physical, emotional and sexual development that occurs during puberty.
- Identify at least two reasons teens have sex, the consequences of sex and strategies for reducing those consequences.

MODULE PREVIEW

The second module: (1) helps students explore the changes that occur during adolescence; and (2) explores pressures to engage in sexual activities.

STRATEGIES/METHODS

- DVD Viewing
- Group Discussion
- Brainstorming

MATERIALS NEEDED — INCLUDED IN IMPLEMENTATION KIT

- *Body Changes* poster
- Optional posters:
  - » *Female Body—Outside*
  - » *Female Body—Inside*
  - » *Male Body—Inside*
- DVD: *The Subject Is Puberty* (Abstinence Version)

MATERIALS NEEDED — NOT INCLUDED IN IMPLEMENTATION KIT

- Markers
- Masking tape
- Monitor and DVD player
- Pre-labeled newsprint:
  - » *Why Some Young People Have Sex*
  - » *Consequences of Sex*
  - » *Proud and Responsible Prevention Strategies*

PREPARATION NEEDED

1. Label all of the newsprint charts as listed under Materials.

2. Hang the poster and pre-labeled newsprint charts in the order they will be used. Fold and tape the charts so the titles remain covered by the bottom half of the sheet until you use them.

3. Make sure *The Subject Is Puberty* DVD is set up and ready to play.

4. Prepare to review and define the following terms (definitions in the glossary) throughout the lesson as needed:

» acne	» hips	» sexual attraction
» anus	» hormones	» sexually active
» body/pubic hair	» labia	» sperm
» breasts	» menstrual cycle (period)	» tampon
» cervix	» menstruation	» testicles
» clitoris	» muscles	» testosterone
» consequences	» ovaries	» urethra
» egg	» penis	» uterus
» estrogen	» pituitary gland	» vagina
» fallopian tube	» puberty	» vaginal opening
» fertilized egg	» pubic bone	» voice
» gender	» scrotum	» vulva
» genitals	» scrotum	» womb

Making a Difference! For Youth with Cognitive Impairments

5. Be prepared to review key concepts from the first module.

INSTRUCTIONAL TIME: 45–60 minutes

ACTIVITY	MINUTES NEEDED
Pre-Activity: Key Concept Review	5
A. Puberty and Adolescent Sexual Development	30–40
B. Brainstorming About Young People and Sex	10–15

PREPARING FOR THE ACTIVITY

RATIONALE

Providing students with a brief review of key topics discussed in the previous module will reinforce their learning, prime them for new learning and help transition to the concepts in the upcoming module.

MATERIALS

None

TIME

5 minutes

PROCEDURE

1. Begin by writing the names of key concepts learned in the last module on the board:

   » *Making a Difference!* Program
   This program is about helping you avoid unplanned pregnancy and diseases that are transmitted sexually.

   » Group Agreements
   Guidelines that will help the group feel safe and comfortable sharing during the program.

   » Being Proud and Responsible
   Valuing yourself and making healthy choices, such as abstinence.

   » Abstinence
   Choosing not to do any sexual behaviors that could cause pregnancy or spread disease.

   » Goals and Obstacles
   Goals are things people want to accomplish, and obstacles are things that make goals harder to achieve, such as pregnancy or STDs from sexual activity.

2. Ask for a volunteer to explain what one of the concepts means.

3. Clarify concept if needed.

4. Check for understanding with a few other students. Repeat process with the remaining concepts.

5. Define any terms from this module that you expect your students will need to have defined before beginning the lesson. Terms may include:

<table>
<tr><td>» acne</td><td>» hips</td><td>» sexually active</td></tr>
<tr><td>» anus</td><td>» hormones</td><td>» sperm</td></tr>
<tr><td>» body/pubic hair</td><td>» labia</td><td>» tampon</td></tr>
<tr><td>» breasts</td><td>» menstrual cycle (period)</td><td>» testicles</td></tr>
<tr><td>» cervix</td><td></td><td>» testosterone</td></tr>
<tr><td>» clitoris</td><td>» menstruation</td><td>» urethra</td></tr>
<tr><td>» consequences</td><td>» muscles</td><td>» uterus</td></tr>
<tr><td>» egg</td><td>» ovaries</td><td>» vagina</td></tr>
<tr><td>» estrogen</td><td>» penis</td><td>» vaginal opening</td></tr>
<tr><td>» fallopian tube</td><td>» pituitary gland</td><td>» voice</td></tr>
<tr><td>» fertilized egg</td><td>» puberty</td><td>» vulva</td></tr>
<tr><td>» gender</td><td>» pubic bone</td><td>» womb</td></tr>
<tr><td>» genitals</td><td>» scrotum</td><td></td></tr>
<tr><td></td><td>» sexual attraction</td><td></td></tr>
</table>

6. Explain to students that last time they learned that making proud and responsible choices will help them reach their goals. Today they are going to learn about puberty and how it changes their bodies. Then they will brainstorm why people choose to have sex, and the consequences that can happen when people become sexually active.

PREPARING FOR THE ACTIVITY

RATIONALE

Learning more about the physical and emotional changes of puberty and basic information about anatomy and reproduction helps students develop more confidence in their own knowledge, which can enhance their decision-making skills.

ACTIVITY LEARNING OBJECTIVE

- Identify the physical, emotional and sexual development that occurs during puberty.

MATERIALS

- Monitor and DVD player
- DVD: *The Subject Is Puberty*
- *Body Changes* poster
- Optional posters:
  - » *Female Body—Outside*
  - » *Female Body—Inside*
  - » *Male Body—Inside*

TIME

30–40 minutes

PROCEDURE

1a. Tell the group that they are going to watch a DVD about puberty and sexual development. Explain that puberty is the time when young peoples' bodies change to become adult bodies, and the DVD will go over what types of changes happen.

1b. Tell students the DVD is broken up into 4 parts. Tell them after each part you will ask the class some questions about what they just saw.

2a. Show Part 1: Introduction. While the DVD is playing, post the *Body Changes* poster.

2b. Pause at the end of the segment, 4:16. Process the segment by asking these questions:

- When does puberty usually begin?

- What types of changes happen during puberty?

3. Show Part 2: Hormonal Changes in Boys. Pause at the end of the segment, 6:50. Process the segment by asking:

- What are the physical changes of puberty for boys?

If students have trouble answering the question, review some of the changes listed on the poster.

4. Show Part 3: Hormonal Changes in Girls. Pause at the end of the segment, 11:08. Process the segment by asking:

> • **What are the physical changes of puberty for girls?**

If students have trouble answering the question, review some of the changes listed on the poster.

5. Show Part 4: Review and Sexual Attraction. At the end of the segment, process by asking:

> • **What are some of the emotional changes teenagers go through during puberty?**

Answers could include:

» Need to make own decisions and have more say in their lives

» Desire to be accepted by peers

» Rebelling against those that make the rules

» Emotional mood swings

» Sometimes wanting to be alone or only with particular people

» Feelings about gender expectations

» Feeling unsure, nervous or excited about changes

» Hopes and dreams for the future

» Developing attractions toward other people

» Development of sexual feelings

6. After the DVD, ask students if they have any questions about the information presented.

7. Summarize as follows,

KEY MESSAGE:

Puberty is when people may first have sexual feelings.

These sexual feelings may cause physical and emotional reactions.

Sexual feelings are normal.

Having sexual feelings does not mean you have to have sex.

Puberty is when many young people begin to have sexual feelings. Sexual feelings can cause physical reactions, such as sweaty palms, faster heartbeat, erections (when the penis becomes hard and stands out away from the body) and warm or tingly sensations in the vulva or genital area. Sexual feelings also cause emotional reactions, such as thinking about the person you're attracted to, feeling happy or confused, or wanting to spend time with that person.

Sexual feelings are normal. Not everyone experiences sexual feelings, but when people do, these feelings can be strong and confusing. It's what you do about them that's important! Sometimes young people act on these feelings without thinking things through. The proud and responsible thing to do is to take time to get to know and understand your feelings. You do not have to have sex just because you're experiencing sexual feelings.

ACTIVITY B

BRAINSTORMING ABOUT YOUNG PEOPLE AND SEX

PREPARING FOR THE ACTIVITY

RATIONALE

By exploring issues about youth and sex, students become more aware of the pressures they face and the choices they may have to make. It gives the facilitator more information about the thoughts and feelings of the students and helps the students learn more about the focus of the program.

ACTIVITY LEARNING OBJECTIVE

- Identify at least two reasons teens have sex, the consequences of sex and strategies for reducing those consequences.

MATERIALS

- Pre-labeled newsprint (examples on right):
  - » *Why Some Young People Have Sex*
  - » *Consequences of Sex*
  - » *Proud and Responsible Prevention Strategies*
- Markers
- Masking tape

TIME

10–15 minutes

PROCEDURE

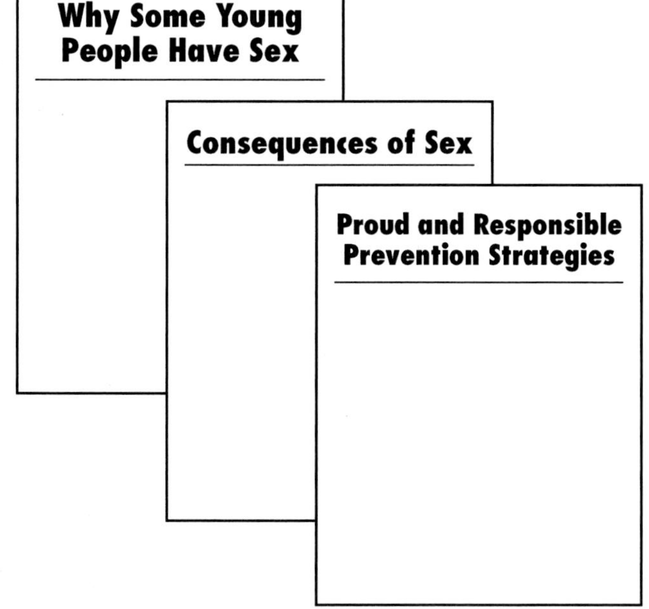

FACILITATOR'S NOTE

As you facilitate this activity and the entire program, keep in mind that for some youth pregnancy and parenting are intentional. The reasons are complex. There may be family, cultural and community influences—in some families, cultures and communities, young parenthood is prized and has been modeled. Some youth place high value on parenthood because they see it as a realistic life option when they don't see options such as post-secondary education and/or a career

(continued)

1. For this activity, use the pre-labeled newsprint (folded so that the titles are covered by the bottom half of the newsprint). Unfold the newsprint sheets one at a time, as needed.

2. Before introducing the activity, remind students that brainstorming is saying whatever comes to mind about a particular issue or question.

FACILITATOR'S NOTE

If students have challenges with brainstorming, offer some suggestions as examples. Solicit ideas from individuals in the group, or, if students are still struggling, present ideas for them to agree or disagree with.

3. Unfold the first sheet of newsprint titled *Why Some Young People Have Sex*, and ask students why they think some young people their age would choose to have sex.

FACILITATOR'S NOTE

If necessary, remind students that sex is sexual touching involving: (1) putting a penis into a vagina (vaginal sex); (2) putting a mouth on another person's penis, vagina or anus (oral sex); or (3) putting a penis into another person's anus (anal sex).

The responses should include the following:

- » To get or keep a boyfriend/girlfriend/ partner or because partner expects it
- » To get attention or affection
- » Loneliness
- » For pleasure or sexual release
- » To have fun
- » To feel loved or needed
- » To feel more grown up
- » Problems at home/living situation
- » To be popular
- » See it on TV or in the movies

» To get back at parents

» Forced

» To have a baby

» To increase status in peer group

» To fit in with peer group

» Low self-esteem

» To satisfy curiosity

» To prove masculinity/femininity

» To express feelings of love or affection to a partner

4. Write all students' comments, or ideas from you that students agreed with, on the newsprint.

5. Compliment their good ideas.

6. Summarize as follows,

KEY MESSAGE:

There are many reasons young people might have sex, but there are also many good reasons to choose abstinence, including that having sex could make it harder to achieve your goals.

As we can see, there are many reasons young people might have sex. But there are also many good reasons for them to choose abstinence and wait to have sex. The consequences of having sex at a young age could make it harder to accomplish their goals for the future.

FACILITATOR'S NOTE

You may choose to reintroduce the *Goals and Obstacles* newsprint list from Module 1 to remind students of the goals that having sex could make harder to achieve.

7. Tell students now you're going to look at some of the possible consequences of sex. Unfold the next newsprint, *Consequences of Sex*.

8. Ask the group to name some of the consequences of sex.

Be sure to include:

» Pregnancy

» HIV

» STDs

 Making a Difference! For Youth with Cognitive Impairments

9.   Write all of their comments on the newsprint.

Students may also mention positive consequences of having sex, such as feeling closer to a partner or experiencing pleasure. You can relate these to some of the reasons teens choose to have sex, while also emphasizing that abstinence can help them avoid the consequences that could have a negative impact on their future goals.

10.   Compliment the group on how much they know.

11.   Next, unfold the newsprint titled *Proud and Responsible Prevention Strategies.*

12.   Have students list ways to prevent the negative consequences of sex.

13.   Write all students' comments on the newsprint. Emphasize that abstaining from sex is the surest way to prevent pregnancy and sexually transmitted diseases.

14.   Compliment the group on how much they know.

15.   Point to their lists and summarize by saying,

KEY MESSAGE:

While there are many reasons young people may have sex, it has many possible consequences. Using a proud and responsible prevention strategy such as abstinence will help you avoid the negative consequences of sex.

As we can see by your lists, there are many reasons young people have sex. We can also see there are many consequences of having sex. Yet, there are some proud and responsible strategies for preventing those consequences. You did a great job generating your lists. Throughout our lessons together we will be looking at many of these issues more closely.

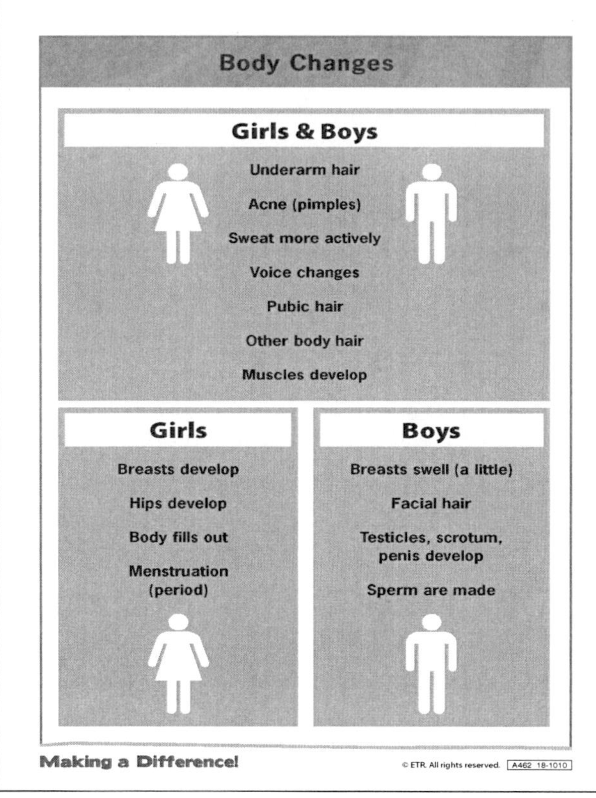

Poster

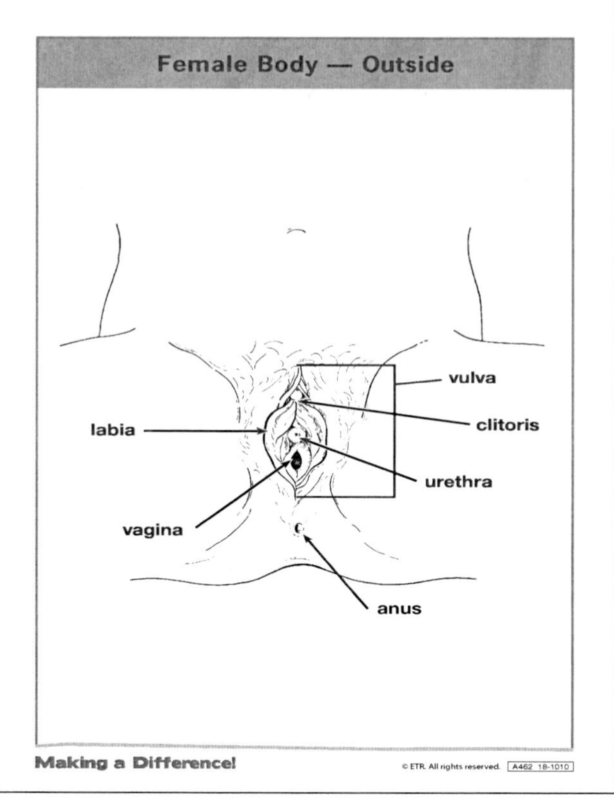

Poster

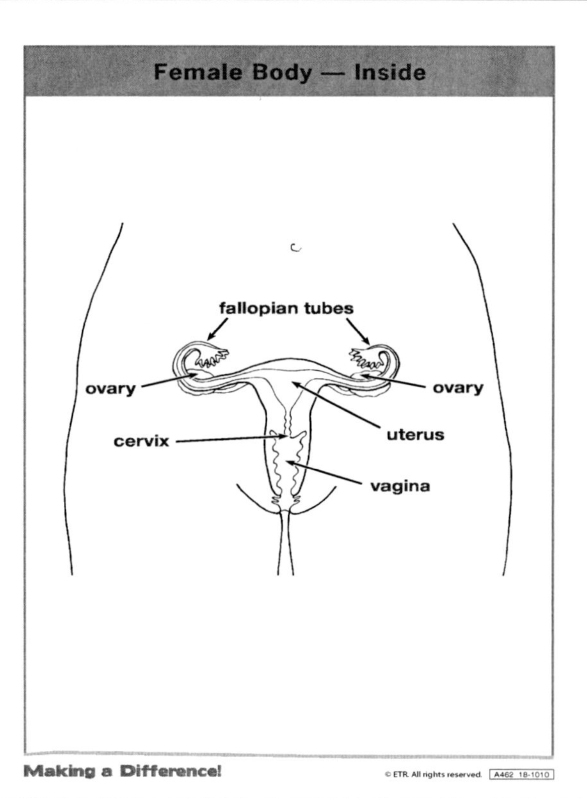

Poster

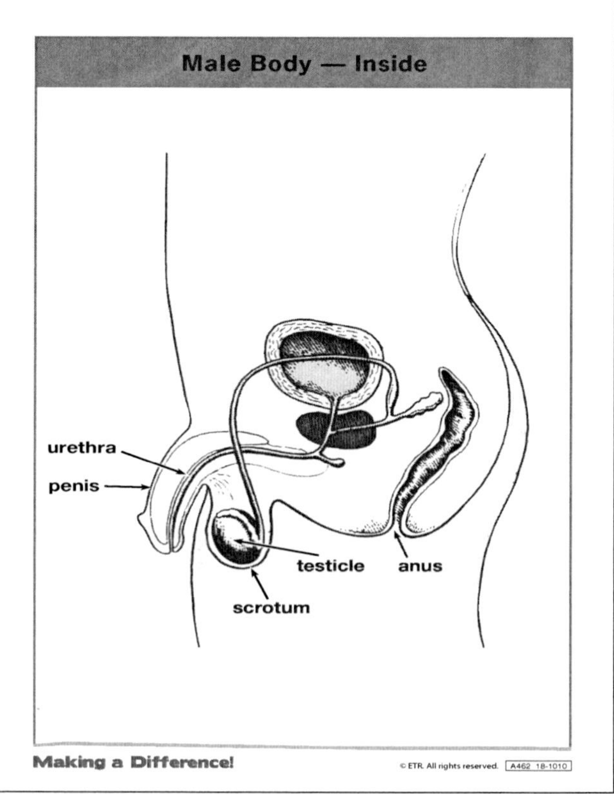

Poster

 Making a Difference! For Youth with Cognitive Impairments

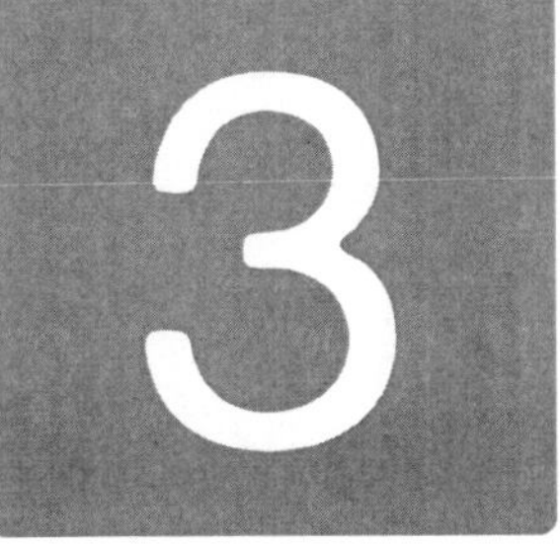

UNDERSTANDING ABSTINENCE

GOALS

The goals of this module are to:

- Review information about why young people have sex.
- Increase students' awareness of the pressures to become involved in sexual activity.
- Increase students' awareness of the benefits of abstinence.
- Use information about self-esteem and peer pressure to help students begin to understand the need to practice abstinence.

LEARNING OBJECTIVES

After completing this module, students will be able to:

- Identify sexual pressures.
- Identify the sexual behaviors to avoid when practicing abstinence.
- Identify some of the benefits of abstinence.
- Identify and name at least five positive characteristics about themselves.
- Explain how self-esteem affects decision making.

MODULE PREVIEW

The third module: (1) explores the pressures to engage in sexual activities; (2) examines alternative ways to express sexual feelings; and (3) encourages students to think about their choices and how their self-esteem might affect those choices.

STRATEGIES/METHODS

- Group Discussion
- Brainstorming

MATERIALS NEEDED — INCLUDED IN IMPLEMENTATION KIT

- *How Do People Express Their Sexual Feelings?* poster
- *Seeing the Positive* handout

MATERIALS NEEDED — NOT INCLUDED IN IMPLEMENTATION KIT

- Markers
- Masking tape
- Blank index cards
- Pre-labeled newsprint:
  - » *Goals* (from Module 1)
  - » *Why Some Young People Have Sex* (from Module 2)
  - » *Benefits of Sex/Abstinence*

PREPARATION NEEDED

1. Label all of the newsprint charts as listed under Materials.

2. Hang the poster and pre-labeled newsprint charts in the order they will be used. Fold and tape the new chart so the title remains covered by the bottom half of the sheet until you use it.

3. Prepare to review and define the following terms (definitions in the glossary) throughout the lesson as needed:

   - » anal sex
   - » bisexual
   - » cuddling
   - » French kiss
   - » gay
   - » genital contact
   - » intercourse
   - » lesbian
   - » masturbation
   - » oral sex
   - » pressure
   - » sexual fantasy
   - » sexual orientation
   - » touching
   - » vaginal sex

4. Be prepared to review key concepts from the second module.

INSTRUCTIONAL TIME: 45–60 minutes

ACTIVITY	MINUTES NEEDED
Pre-Activity: Key Concept Review	5
A. Why Some Young People Have Sex	10
B. How Do People Express Their Sexual Feelings? What Is Abstinence?	10–15
C. Benefits of Sex/Benefits of Abstinence	10–15
D. Seeing the Positive in Yourself	10–15

Making a Difference! For Youth with Cognitive Impairments

PREPARING FOR THE ACTIVITY

RATIONALE

Providing students with a brief review of key topics discussed in the previous module will reinforce their learning, prime them for new learning and help transition to the concepts in the upcoming module.

MATERIALS

Group Agreements

TIME

5 minutes

PROCEDURE

1. Begin by writing the names of key concepts learned in the previous module on the board:

   » Goals and Obstacles
   Goals are things people want to accomplish, and obstacles are things that make goals harder to achieve, such as pregnancy or STDs from sexual activity.

   » Consequences of Sex
   May include pregnancy, STDs or HIV.

2. Ask for a volunteer to explain what one of the concepts means.

3. Clarify concept if needed.

4. Check for understanding with a few other students. Repeat process with the remaining concept.

5. Define any terms from this module that you expect your students will need to have defined before beginning the lesson. Terms may include:

» anal sex	» genital contact	» pressure
» bisexual	» intercourse	» sexual fantasy
» cuddling	» lesbian	» sexual orientation
» French kiss	» masturbation	» touching
» gay	» oral sex	» vaginal sex

6. Tell students that last time the group focused on why young people choose to have sex, and the consequences that can happen when people become sexually active. This time they will learn about different ways people can express their sexual feelings, and the benefits of abstinence.

Making a Difference! For Youth with Cognitive Impairments

WHY SOME YOUNG PEOPLE HAVE SEX

PREPARING FOR THE ACTIVITY

RATIONALE

Exploring the various reasons young people engage in sexual intercourse will help students recognize poor reasons for having sexual intercourse.

ACTIVITY LEARNING OBJECTIVES

- Identify sexual pressures.
- Identify some of the benefits of abstinence.

MATERIALS

- Newsprint from past modules:
  - » *Goals* (from Module 1)
  - » *Why Some Young People Have Sex* (from Module 2)

TIME

10 minutes

PROCEDURE

1. Post the *Goals* and *Why Some Young People Have Sex* newsprint lists from Modules 1 and 2.

2. Remind students of the *Why Some Young People Have Sex* list they brainstormed earlier, and ask if they would like to add anything to the list.

    The list may include:

    - » To get or keep a boyfriend/girlfriend/ partner or because partner expects it
    - » Loneliness
    - » For pleasure or sexual release
    - » To feel loved or needed
    - » To have fun
    - » Problems at home/ living situation
    - » To feel more grown up
    - » To be popular
    - » See it on TV or in the movies

» To get back at parents

» To have a baby

» Forced

» To fit in with peer group

» To increase status in peer group

» To satisfy curiosity

» Low self-esteem

» To express feelings of love or affection to a partner

» To prove masculinity/femininity

» To get attention or affection

FACILITATOR'S NOTE

Stress that when young people have sex for reasons such as "to get or keep a boyfriend or girlfriend" or "to get back at parents," they usually end up hurting themselves.

3a.	Ask the group if there are any reasons on the list that they would risk their future or life for. (Most students will respond "no.")

3b.	Ask how having sexual intercourse might make it more difficult to achieve their goals. Point to the Goals list as students answer. Elicit responses about how pregnancy and sexually transmitted diseases could affect each of these goals.

FACILITATOR'S NOTE

If students have challenges generating ideas on their own, make some example suggestions, then solicit ideas from individuals in the group.

3c.	Next, have the group imagine that some sexually active young people decided to stop having sexual intercourse because it wasn't the best choice for them right now.

Ask how these young people might benefit from that decision.

Encourage the group to see that these young people would be able to focus more on achieving their goals if they didn't have to worry about pregnancy or disease.

Making a Difference! For Youth with Cognitive Impairments

4.   Summarize as follows,

KEY MESSAGE:

While there are many
reasons young people may
have sex, the consequences,
such as pregnancy or
STDs, can get in the way of
your goals. Stay focused
on your goals and choose
abstinence to avoid STDs and
pregnancy.

There are many reasons young people might choose
to have sex. But there are even better reasons to
wait to have sex. The consequences of having sex
can sometimes get in the way of your goals, and
include unplanned pregnancy and STDs. The proud
and responsible thing to do is to stay focused on
achieving your goals and choose to be abstinent (not
have sex) at this time in your life.

PREPARING FOR THE ACTIVITY

RATIONALE

Understanding that there are many behaviors that express sexual feelings helps students choose those that do not result in pregnancy or sexually transmitted disease.

ACTIVITY LEARNING OBJECTIVE

• Identify the sexual behaviors to avoid when practicing abstinence.

MATERIALS

• Masking tape

• *How Do People Express Their Sexual Feelings?* poster

TIME

10–15 minutes

PROCEDURE

1. Have students list some of the ways people express their sexual feelings to themselves or other people.

2. Elicit as many answers as you can.

   Answers may include:

» talking	» sexual fantasy	» vaginal sex
» caressing	» touching	» massage
» hugging	» touching each other's genitals	» anal sex
» cuddling		» masturbation
» holding hands	» saying "I like you"	
» grinding	» oral sex	
» kissing	» dancing	

3. Display the *How Do People Express Their Sexual Feelings?* poster.

4a. Before moving on, explain to the group that it's important to understand that people have different sexual orientations, meaning who they feel sexual attraction for.

4b. Explain that when a person is only attracted to people of the opposite sex (i.e., a male and a female), their sexual orientation is often called "straight." Explain that the sexual orientation "gay" refers to when a person is only attracted to people of the same sex (i.e., two males or two females), and "lesbian" refers to when a female is only attracted to other females. Finally, explain that when a person is attracted to people of either sex, their sexual orientation is known as "bisexual."

4c. Clarify that people may express their sexual feelings with people of a different sex than them, or with people of the same sex. Explain that when people of the same sex have sex, a pregnancy will not happen, but they could still get an STD.

5. Discuss each item on the *How Do People Express Their Sexual Feelings?* poster by asking students whether or not the behavior could result in pregnancy or a sexually transmitted disease. Be sure to identify ALL behaviors that may involve an exchange of blood, semen, vaginal secretions or rectal fluids, as well as skin-to-skin genital contact or touching. (Students may suggest behaviors besides oral, anal and vaginal intercourse that can transmit disease).

HOW DO PEOPLE EXPRESS THEIR SEXUAL FEELINGS?

Sexual behaviors that can result in pregnancy or sexually transmitted disease are followed by the word yes.

- talking—no
- hugging—no
- holding hands—no
- kissing—no (closed mouth); very slight risk for STD with deep "French" kissing
- touching—no
- touching each other's genitals—yes (slight risk for STD)
- saying "I like you"—no
- dancing—no
- massage—no
- masturbation—no (as long as there is no skin-to-skin genital contact)
- caressing—no
- cuddling—no
- grinding—no
- sexual fantasy—no
- oral sex—yes (STD)
- vaginal sex—yes (STD, pregnancy)
- anal sex—yes (STD)

Making a Difference! For Youth with Cognitive Impairments

6a. Have students brainstorm why people might not want to engage in some or all of these behaviors.

Answers may include:

> » Behavior may not feel good or be appealing.
>
> » Behavior might be risky.
>
> » A person might have religious or moral objections to certain behaviors.

6b. Ask students how they let others know what they are willing and not willing to do.

6c. Next, brainstorm the best time to let others know what they are willing and not willing to do.

Answers may include:

> » People need to talk about their limits with their partners.
>
> » They need to tell them before any touching or other sexual contact occurs.

7. Next, ask students what abstinence is.

8. Most students will reply that abstinence means no sex at all. Clarify this by asking which behaviors in particular people should avoid if they are practicing abstinence, and why.

(continued)

- Certain STDs (herpes, syphilis, HPV) can also be transmitted by skin-to-skin genital contact or touching.

- Any behavior that introduces semen into the vagina or onto the vulva can lead to pregnancy.

- Behaviors that do not involve any of these risks may be good ways to express feelings to another person.

9a. Ask the group if they believe that couples who practice abstinence can still share their thoughts and feelings with one another.

9b. Ask the group if they believe that couples who practice abstinence can experience love.

9c. Ask the group if they believe that couples who practice abstinence still build a strong and long-lasting relationship.

10. Summarize as follows,

KEY MESSAGE:

People can express sexual feelings in many ways other than sex. Some ways of expressing sexual feelings are safe, but others can lead to pregnancy or STDs. Abstinence can eliminate risk of STDs and pregnancy.

You can clearly see that sexual expression is not just about having sex. People can express themselves sexually with a wide range of behaviors.

Some of these behaviors are safe and will not lead to pregnancy or STDs, but others are not.

Abstinence—not having vaginal, oral or anal sex and avoiding skin-to-skin genital touching—is the SAFEST and most effective way to prevent an unintended pregnancy and avoid getting an STD. It is a proud and responsible thing to do.

Making a Difference! For Youth with Cognitive Impairments

PREPARING FOR THE ACTIVITY

RATIONALE

Helping students explore the various reasons young people choose not to engage in sexual intercourse and what the benefits of abstinence can be allows them to identify that abstinence is a viable and healthy choice.

ACTIVITY LEARNING OBJECTIVE

• Identify some of the benefits of abstinence.

MATERIALS

• Pre-labeled newsprint:

  » *Benefits of Sex/ Abstinence*

• Markers

TIME

10–15 minutes

Benefits of	
Sex	**Abstinence**

PROCEDURE

1. Hang the *Benefits of Sex/Abstinence* newsprint on the wall.

FACILITATOR'S NOTE

You may have to help the group by prompting them with some of the answers, especially for the benefits of abstinence. Help them but don't give them all the answers. Encourage them to think.

2a. Remind students that the last activity included brainstorms on why young people have sex, and how people can express their sexual feelings.

2b. Ask what young people gain by having sex. Have the group brainstorm the benefits of sex.

3.   Write their answers on the newsprint under the "Sex" column.

      Answers may include:
      » Expression of love
      » Having a baby
      » Sexual release
      » Sense of maturity
      » Revenge
      » Trade for favors, money or drugs
      » Popularity

4.   **Next, ask what young people gain by waiting to have sex or deciding to stop having sex. Have the group brainstorm the benefits of abstinence.**

      Elicit such answers as:
      » Avoid getting pregnant or causing a pregnancy if you're not ready
      » Avoid STDs, including HIV
      » Don't have to worry about parents finding out
      » Avoid emotional or physical pain or discomfort
      » Uphold religious and cultural beliefs
      » Keep focus on achieving future goals
      » Sex may feel better if you wait until you are physically, emotionally and mentally ready
      » Keep focus on finishing school
      » Won't have to worry about raising a child
      » Have time to build a strong relationship before having sex
      » Find out who wants you, and who just wants sex
      » Explore sexual feelings without risking pregnancy or an STD
      » Feel good about making a choice that can keep you safe

5.   **The benefits of abstinence list will probably be longer than the benefits of sex list. Be sure to elicit enough answers to ensure this is the case.**

6a.   **Have students identify differences between the two lists.**

 Making a Difference! For Youth with Cognitive Impairments

6b. Ask the group to brainstorm why these differences exist.

7. Reinforce the benefits of not having sex by asking each student to finish the following sentence:

If I wait to have sex, I will be able to ____________________.

8. Summarize as follows,

KEY MESSAGE:

Sexual activity may lead to pregnancy or STDs and can make it harder to reach your goals.

Young people who choose to have sex may end up dealing with an unintended pregnancy, or get infected with an STD, which can be obstacles to achieving some of their goals.

ACTIVITY

D

SEEING THE POSITIVE IN YOURSELF

PREPARING FOR THE ACTIVITY

RATIONALE

Encouraging students to value themselves and think about their choices will increase the likelihood that they will make good decisions.

ACTIVITY LEARNING OBJECTIVES

- Identify and name at least five positive characteristics about themselves.
- Explain how self-esteem affects decision making.

MATERIALS

- *Seeing the Positive* handout
- Pencils/pens

TIME

10–15 minutes

PROCEDURE

1a. Tell students that now the group will focus on how people make sexual choices. Tell them that some people think self-esteem plays a major role in making sexual choices.

1b. Ask students what self-esteem is.

> **Possible answers:**
>
> » The way you feel about yourself.
>
> » How much you like yourself and respect yourself.
>
> » Your belief in the good things about yourself.

2a. Distribute the *Seeing the Positive* handout.

Making a Difference! For Youth with Cognitive Impairments

2b. Ask students to think about all the good things they know about themselves (even things that other people might not know).

2c. Have students circle the good things about themselves on the worksheet.

FACILITATOR'S NOTE

If some of your students find reading challenging, read the words out loud before they start completing the worksheet. Define any words students don't understand.

3.   Allow a few minutes to complete the worksheet. Then ask students, one at a time, to share two good things about themselves.

FACILITATOR'S NOTE

Emphasize the importance of seeing good qualities in ourselves and others.

4.   Ask students how having high or low self-esteem can affect someone's ability to make good decisions.

Answers should include:

» If you have high self-esteem, you won't let anything stand in the way of achieving your goals.

» If you have low self-esteem, you might allow yourself to be pressured into things you don't really want to do, such as having sexual intercourse.

FACILITATOR'S NOTE

If students have challenges generating ideas on their own, make some suggestions to begin the discussion.

5.   Read the following scenarios to the group. Ask students to identify which situations show people with high self-esteem, and which show people with low self-esteem. Ask students to explain why.

1. A person makes a decision based on what feels right, even when friends choose something else. Does this person have high or low self-esteem? Why? **(High)**

2. Someone who feels unattractive decides to have sex to get attention from other people. Does this person have high or low self-esteem? Why? **(Low)**

3. A person respects a partner's decision to wait to have sexual intercourse. Does this person have high or low self-esteem? Why? **(High)**

4. A person pressures someone into sexual behaviors that other person doesn't want to do, then brags about it to friends. Does this person have high or low self-esteem? Why? **(Low)**

5. A person decides not to have oral, anal or vaginal sex. Does this person have high or low self-esteem? Why? **(High)**

FACILITATOR'S NOTE

To get all students engaged in the activity, you can instruct them to use a thumbs-up sign for high self-esteem and a thumbs-down for low self-esteem.

6. Summarize by saying,

KEY MESSAGE:

Self-esteem can affect people's decisions about sex. When you have high self-esteem and feel good about yourself, you make healthy choices, such as practicing abstinence, that help you reach your goals.

Self-esteem affects the sexual choices people make, including whether they engage in sex. When you feel good about yourself, you make healthy sexual decisions, such as practicing abstinence, that will help protect your future and make it possible to reach your goals.

Making a Difference! For Youth with Cognitive Impairments

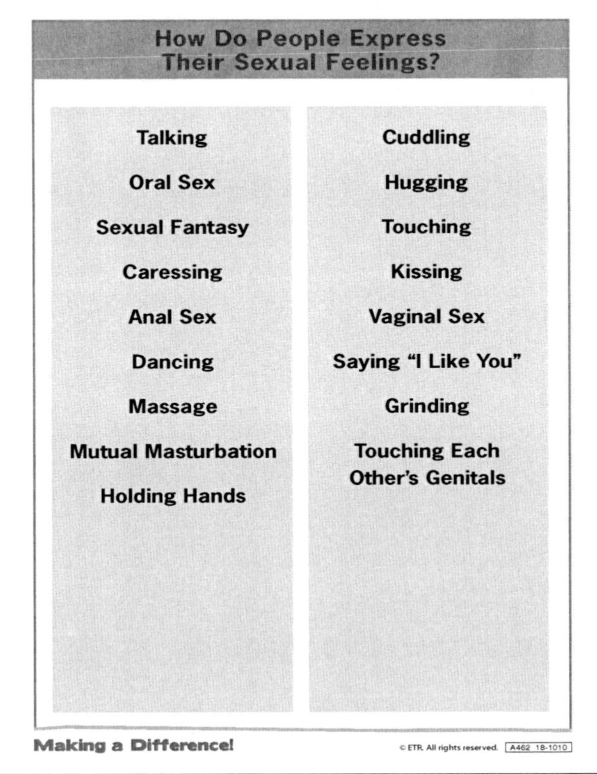

Poster

Seeing the Positive

Handout

Circle at least **five** qualities that you think best describe you.

- Creative
- Attractive
- Sensitive
- Responsible
- Caring
- Brave
- Thankful
- Funny

- Healthy
- Strong
- Hard-working
- Musical
- Honest
- Loyal
- Friendly

- Thoughtful
- Loving
- Smart
- Athletic
- Patient
- Kind
- Proud

Other good things not listed but true about you:

____

____

____

____

____

Handout

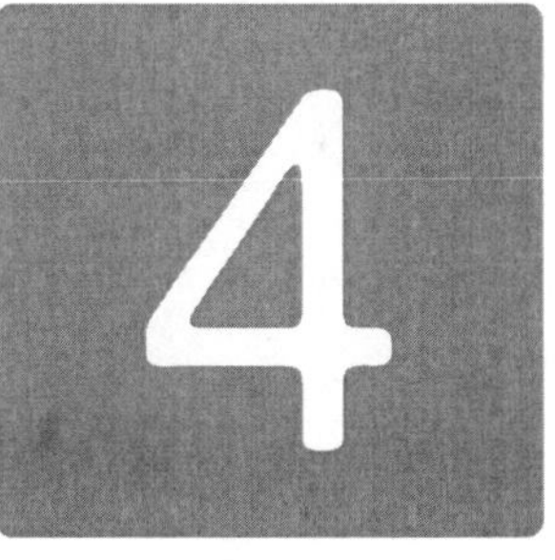

MODULE 4

THE CONSEQUENCES OF SEX: HIV INFECTION

GOALS

The goals of this module are to:

- Increase students' knowledge about HIV/AIDS and HIV risk-associated behavior.

- Help students identify behaviors that place people at risk for contracting sexually transmitted diseases, including HIV.

LEARNING OBJECTIVES

After completing this module, students will be able to:

- Identify the basic facts about HIV and AIDS.

- Identify which behaviors are low risk, high risk and no risk for contracting HIV.

- Identify a person's risk of HIV infection as a result of engaging in various sexual and non-sexual behaviors.

- Identify how HIV infection can be prevented.

MODULE PREVIEW

The fourth module: (1) clarifies myths about the causes, transmission and prevention of HIV and provides the correct information; and (2) helps students identify various behaviors that place them at risk for HIV infection.

STRATEGIES/METHODS

- DVD Viewing
- Group Discussion
- Game
- Brainstorming

MATERIALS NEEDED — INCLUDED IN IMPLEMENTATION KIT

- DVD: *The Subject Is HIV* (Abstinence Version)
- Posters:
    » *HIV/AIDS Review*
    » *Key Words*
- *Risk Continuum* signs
- *Risk Behavior* cards

MATERIALS NEEDED — NOT INCLUDED IN IMPLEMENTATION KIT

- Monitor and DVD player

PREPARATION NEEDED

1. Hang the posters in the order they will be used.

2. Make sure *The Subject Is HIV* DVD is set up and ready to play.

3. Prepare to review and define the following terms (definitions in the glossary) throughout the lesson as needed:

» AIDS	» condom	» monogamous
» body fluids	» disease	» risk behavior
– saliva	» dry kissing	» syndrome
– sweat	» HIV	» virus
– urine	» immune system	
» casual contact	» infection	

4. Be prepared to review key concepts from the third module.

INSTRUCTIONAL TIME: 45–60 minutes

ACTIVITY   MINUTES NEEDED

Pre-Activity: Key Concept Review 5

A. *The Subject Is HIV* **DVD and Discussion** 25–35

B. **HIV Risk Continuum** 15–20

 Making a Difference! For Youth with Cognitive Impairments

KEY CONCEPT REVIEW

PREPARING FOR THE ACTIVITY

RATIONALE

Providing students with a brief review of key topics discussed in the previous module will reinforce their learning, prime them for new learning and help transition to the concepts in the upcoming module.

MATERIALS

None

TIME

5 minutes

PROCEDURE

1. Begin by writing the names of key concepts learned in the last module on the board:

   » Benefits of Abstinence
   Avoiding the consequences of sex, including pregnancy and STDs.

   » Self-esteem
   The way someone feels about themselves. Someone with high self-esteem won't let anything stand in the way of their goals, while someone with low self-esteem may allow themselves to be pressured into things they don't want to do such as having sex.

2. Ask for a volunteer to explain what one of the concepts means.

3. Clarify concept if needed.

4. Check for understanding with a few other students. Repeat process with the remaining concept.

5. **Define any terms from this module that you expect your students will need to have defined before beginning the lesson. Terms may include:**

» AIDS	» condom	» monogamous
» body fluids	» disease	» risk behavior
– saliva	» dry kissing	» syndrome
– sweat	» HIV	» virus
– urine	» immune system	
» casual contact	» infection	

6. **Tell students that last time they learned about making healthy sexual decisions, such as practicing abstinence. This will help protect their future and make it possible to reach their goals. This time they will learn how to protect themselves from the consequences of sex, including HIV.**

Making a Difference! For Youth with Cognitive Impairments

PREPARING FOR THE ACTIVITY

RATIONALE

This activity will help students learn about HIV transmission and AIDS.

ACTIVITY LEARNING OBJECTIVES

- Identify the basic facts about HIV and AIDS.
- Identify how HIV infection can be prevented.

MATERIALS

- Monitor and DVD Player
- DVD: *The Subject Is HIV* (Abstinence Version)
- *HIV/AIDS Review* poster
- *Key Words* poster

TIME

25–35 minutes

PROCEDURE

1. Introduce the DVD called *The Subject Is HIV*, which will discuss HIV/AIDS, what it is, how you can get it and how to prevent infection. Explain to students the DVD is broken up into 3 parts. Tell students that after each part you will ask the class some questions about what they just saw.

FACILITATOR'S NOTE

You may choose to break the DVD up into smaller segments for processing if it would be beneficial to your students.

Before moving on to each segment of the DVD, ask students if they have any questions about the part they just watched.

(continued)

> *(continued)*
>
> Some statistics have changed since the video was produced. In 2016, youth ages 13 to 24 accounted for an estimated 21% of new HIV infections in the United States. The most recent data on young people and HIV can be found at: www.cdc.gov/hiv/group/age/youth/index.html

2a. Show Part 1: Introduction. While the DVD is playing, post the *HIV/AIDS Review* and *Key Words* posters.

2b. Pause at the end of the segment, 6:56. Process the segment by asking these questions:

- **How can a person get HIV/AIDS?**
- **Is there a cure for HIV?**
- **What is the surest way to prevent HIV?**

3. Show Part 2: Talking with Friends. Pause at the end of the segment, 12:28. Process the segment by asking:

- **Why did the girls think it was important to wait to have sex?**
- **What did the boys talk about that convinced Bryan to wait to have sex?**

4. Show Part 3: HIV Positive Individuals and Testing. At the conclusion of the DVD, ask students the questions below:

- **What were the main messages in the DVD?**
- **What do you think the DVD was trying to tell you?**

Answers should include:

- » You can get HIV/AIDS from oral sex, vaginal sex and anal sex.
- » Mothers can give HIV to their babies before birth.
- » You can get HIV from sharing needles.
- » You cannot tell who has HIV by looking.
- » There is no cure for HIV.

Making a Difference! For Youth with Cognitive Impairments

5. Direct the group's attention to the *HIV/AIDS Review* and *Key Words* posters. Ask the group the following questions. Allow students the opportunity to provide answers, and provide them with correct information when necessary. Answer the questions with all the information below.

KEY MESSAGE:

HIV, the virus that causes AIDS, damages the body's immune system. There is no cure for HIV, but there are treatments.

KEY MESSAGE:

AIDS is the stage of HIV when the immune system is very weak. People with AIDS can become very sick from other diseases because their immune system isn't strong.

HIV/AIDS REVIEW POSTER— QUESTIONS AND ANSWERS

What is HIV?

- HIV stands for human immunodeficiency virus. It is the virus that causes AIDS (acquired immunodeficiency syndrome). People who have HIV in their bodies are said to have HIV or to be HIV positive.

- HIV damages the body's immune system, which normally protects the body from disease. The immune system becomes weaker until it can no longer fight off different types of infections.

- There is no cure for HIV, but treatments can be started while the person still feels healthy. With these medicines, people with HIV can lead longer and healthier lives than ever before.

What is AIDS?

- AIDS stands for acquired immunodeficiency syndrome. AIDS is the stage of HIV when the immune system has become very weak and damaged. When this happens, other diseases and infections can enter the body. These are called "opportunistic infections" because they take advantage of the weakened immune system.

(continued)

KEY MESSAGE:

People can get HIV through unprotected sex or sharing needles. Babies can get HIV from their mothers before or during birth.

KEY MESSAGE:

Body fluids that can transmit HIV are blood, semen, vaginal and rectal fluids.

KEY MESSAGE:

A person cannot get HIV through touching, hugging, coughing, sneezing, sharing food or utensils, insect bites or toilet seats.

(continued)

HIV/AIDS REVIEW POSTER— QUESTIONS AND ANSWERS

How do people get HIV?

- Through sex. Anyone who has unprotected vaginal or anal sex with someone who has HIV can get HIV. There is also some risk of transmission through oral sex, but it is much lower.

- By sharing needles for injecting drugs, vitamins, steroids or hormones, or for tattooing, piercing or any other reason.

- From mother to child either before or during birth. In a few cases HIV has been passed from mother to child through breastfeeding. A pregnant woman with HIV can take medicines to greatly lower the risk of her baby being born with HIV.

What common body fluids can transmit HIV?

- HIV is found in the blood, semen and vaginal and rectal fluids of someone with HIV. It is passed from person to person through these body fluids.

How is HIV not transmitted?

- HIV is not transmitted by casual, day-to-day contact between people. It is not transmitted through the air. It must get inside the body to infect a person.

- People can't get HIV from:
    - touching, coughing or sneezing
    - toilet seats, eating utensils, swimming pools, water fountains, door knobs or phones
    - casual contact such as hugging, dry kissing or sharing food
    - donating blood
    - tears, saliva, sweat or urine
    - mosquitoes or other insects   *(continued)*

Making a Difference! For Youth with Cognitive Impairments

KEY MESSAGE:

People are at risk for HIV if
they have unprotected sex or
if they share needles.

KEY MESSAGE:

Not having sex or sharing
needles can prevent you
from getting HIV.

(continued)

Who is at risk?

- It is what people do, not who they are, that puts
  them at risk for HIV. People are at risk for HIV if:
  - They have sex with someone who's had other
    partners.
  - They have sex without using a latex condom or
    other protection.
  - They share needles or syringes to inject drugs,
    or have sex with someone who has.
  - They share needles or other sharp objects for
    tattooing, piercing or any other reason.

How can you prevent HIV?

- Don't have sex. This includes vaginal, anal and
  oral sex.

- Never inject drugs or share needles for any reason.

FACILITATOR'S NOTE

Some students may correctly assert that condoms can be used to reduce the risk of sexually
transmitted diseases, including HIV. Acknowledge that this is true. Correctly using condoms and
other forms of protection, such as dental dams, every time can reduce the risk of STDs, including
HIV and viral hepatitis. Emphasize, however, that abstinence is the surest and most effective way
to eliminate the possibility of sexually transmitted diseases, including HIV. But don't discourage
condom use or provide exaggerated information on failure rates.

6. Next review the following questions using the *Key Words* poster. Ask the following
    questions in a round-robin fashion. Encourage all students to respond. Supplement
    their answers with the information below each question.

KEY MESSAGE:

HIV is the virus that can cause AIDS. It enters the body and damages the immune system. People can live with HIV and remain healthy for many years, though they can still transmit it to others.

KEY MESSAGE:

The immune system is the body's defense against infections. HIV weakens the immune system making it harder to fight off infections.

KEY WORDS POSTER— QUESTIONS AND ANSWERS

How is AIDS different from HIV?

- HIV is the virus that enters the body and damages the immune system. People can live with HIV for years without getting sick. They may look and feel healthy and may not even know they have the virus. People who are taking medicine to treat HIV may be in this stage for several decades, although they can still transmit HIV to others.

- AIDS is the condition that develops as a result of the damage done to the immune system. A person with HIV is diagnosed as having AIDS when their white blood cell count drops below a certain level, or when certain opportunistic infections develop.

What is the immune system?

- The immune system is the body's defense against infections and diseases. When the immune system works as it should, white blood cells patrol the body and attack viruses and bacteria that shouldn't be there.

- HIV attacks white blood cells. As the number of properly working white blood cells decreases, the immune system becomes weaker until it can no longer fight off different types of infections.

- The most common treatments for HIV limit the ability of the virus to reproduce. They help protect the immune system and improve the chances of staying healthy.

(continued)

Making a Difference! For Youth with Cognitive Impairments

What is the test for HIV?

KEY MESSAGE:

HIV is tested with a blood or cheek swab test. These tests check blood or saliva for proteins the body makes in response to HIV.

- The most common type of HIV test looks for HIV antibodies in the body by testing blood or saliva. Antibodies are proteins the body makes in response to a virus. If a person has antibodies for HIV, he or she has HIV and can pass the virus to other people.

- There is also an HIV test that looks for antigens. An antigen is a protein that produces antibodies. HIV antigens can be detected very soon after infection (1–3 weeks) by testing the blood. These tests are more expensive and are not typically used for routine HIV testing. A person who has antigens for HIV has HIV and can pass the virus to other people.

- The PCR (polymerase chain reaction) tests blood for the genetic material of HIV. Blood supplies in most developed countries are screened for HIV using PCR tests. A person who has HIV genetic material has HIV and can pass the virus to other people.

What is the waiting period?

KEY MESSAGE:

The waiting period is the time between when a person gets HIV and when it can be detected with a test. This can be from 2 weeks to 3 months. A person can transmit HIV to others during this time.

- The "waiting period" is the length of time between when a person first gets HIV and when an HIV test can begin to detect signs of the virus in the body. It can be from 2 weeks to 3 months long, depending on what type of test is done. During the window period, even before they know they are infected, people can transmit HIV to others.

(continued)

KEY MESSAGE:

Early HIV treatment can help prevent HIV from progressing and damaging the immune system.

Why is early treatment so important?

- There is no cure for HIV, but anti-retroviral treatments (ART) can be started while the person still feels healthy. If people with HIV remain in medical care and continue to take the medicines to keep low viral loads, they can live long, healthy lives.

7. Conclude the activity by telling students that knowing the basic facts about HIV can help them make a difference and make healthy choices so they can reach their goals.

PREPARING FOR THE ACTIVITY

RATIONALE

Actively identifying the risk level for a variety of sexual and nonsexual behaviors allows students to internalize the information and facilitates learning.

ACTIVITY LEARNING OBJECTIVES

- Identify which behaviors are low risk, high risk and no risk for contracting HIV.
- Identify a person's risk of HIV infection as a result of engaging in various sexual and non-sexual behaviors.
- Identify how HIV infection can be prevented.

MATERIALS

- *Risk Continuum* signs
- *Risk Behavior* cards
- Masking tape

TIME

15–20 minutes

PROCEDURE

1. Tape the *Risk Continuum* signs on the wall or board like the diagram below.

    Unsafe   Be Careful   Safe

FACILITATOR'S NOTE

Alternatively you may choose to designate one side of the room as "Unsafe" and the other as "Safe" and have students move between the sides of the room with "Be Careful" being in the middle.

2a. Remind the group that the last activity reviewed facts about HIV, and that HIV can be prevented if people do not engage in risky sexual behaviors.

2b. Explain that, in this activity, the group will determine how risky certain behaviors are with respect to HIV infection:

- **Unsafe/Red-Light Behaviors** involve contact with blood, semen, vaginal secretions or rectal fluids and can transmit HIV.

- **Be Careful/Yellow-Light Behaviors** are those activities that might pose some danger of transmitting HIV, but from which transmission is less likely to occur.

- **Safe/Green-Light Behaviors** involve no exchange of blood, semen, vaginal secretions or rectal fluids and thus pose no risk of transmitting HIV.

FACILITATOR'S NOTE

Review the behaviors list and define any terms students may not be familiar with such as condom (a thin rubber sheath worn on a penis during sex that helps prevent pregnancy and STD transmission).

3. Shuffle the *Risk Behavior* cards and read the behaviors aloud one at a time. Explain that "sex" in these questions means oral, anal and/or vaginal intercourse.

4. Ask students where they think each card should be placed on the continuum. After each answer, have students explain why they think the behavior belongs under that particular category. Ask if other group members agree. Use this opportunity to clarify misinformation.

5. Once there is agreement about where the *Risk Behavior* card should be placed, ask a student to go tape the card under the correct category.

 Making a Difference! For Youth with Cognitive Impairments

6. Summarize as follows,

KEY MESSAGE:

Some sexual behaviors have more risk of transmitting HIV than others. Risky sexual activity may interfere with goals. Abstinence, or not having sex, can eliminate risk and protect you from HIV.

To protect yourself from HIV infection, it is important to know which behaviors are safe and which are risky. As you can see, there are plenty of behaviors that are Safe or Green Light. People do not need to engage in behaviors that carry a risk of HIV to express themselves sexually. The surest way to protect yourself from HIV and other STDs is to make healthy sexual decisions, such as practicing abstinence.

RISK BEHAVIORS

Vaginal sex — Red Light

Dry kissing — Green Light

Having sex with a person who is having sex with other people — Red Light

Romantic conversation — Green Light

Oral sex of the penis — Yellow/Red Light

Sharing eating utensils or holding hands with someone who has HIV — Green Light

Sharing needles and syringes — Red Light

Anal sex* — Red Light

Self-masturbation — Green Light

Mutual masturbation — Yellow/Green Light
(Green for HIV. There are some STDs [herpes, syphilis, HPV] that can be passed through skin-to-skin contact or genital touching.)

Practicing abstinence — Green Light

Massage — Green Light

Having sex with multiple partners — Red Light

Oral sex of the vulva (female genitals) — Yellow Light

Having sex with a person who shares needles — Red Light

Sexual fantasy — Green Light

Touching someone who has HIV — Green Light

Talking about how you feel and making plans for the future — Green Light

Hugging — Green Light

Having sex with only one person (monogamous) — Green/Yellow/Red Light
(Green if both have never had sex before. If one or both have had other partners, Yellow if use condoms; Red if don't use condoms.)

* Anal sex is a very risky behavior. It is a high risk/red-light behavior without a condom. With a condom, it is still more risky than vaginal sex—somewhere between yellow and red. For safety reasons, it's best to avoid anal sex.

Making a Difference! For Youth with Cognitive Impairments

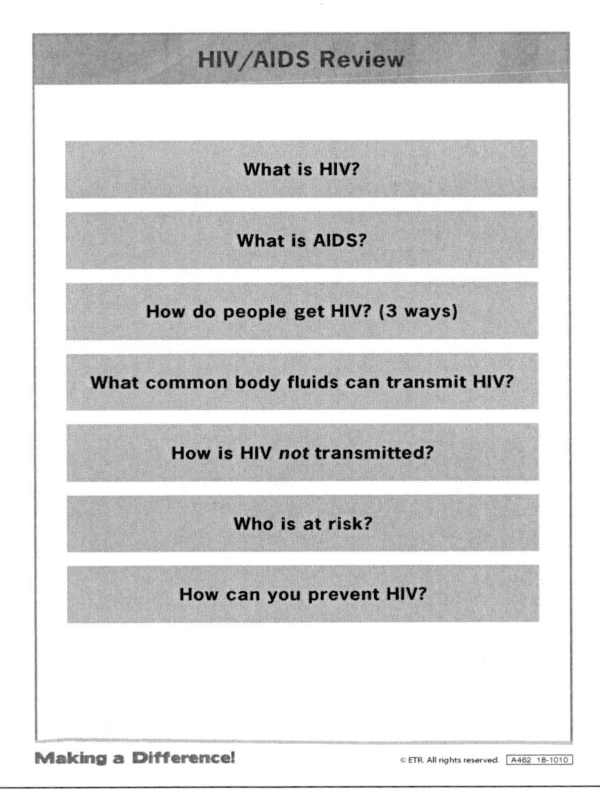

Poster

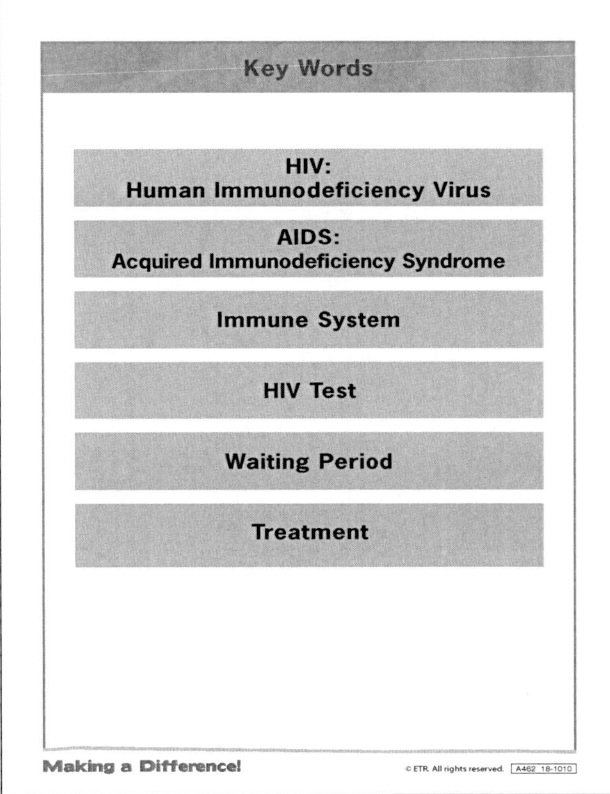

Poster

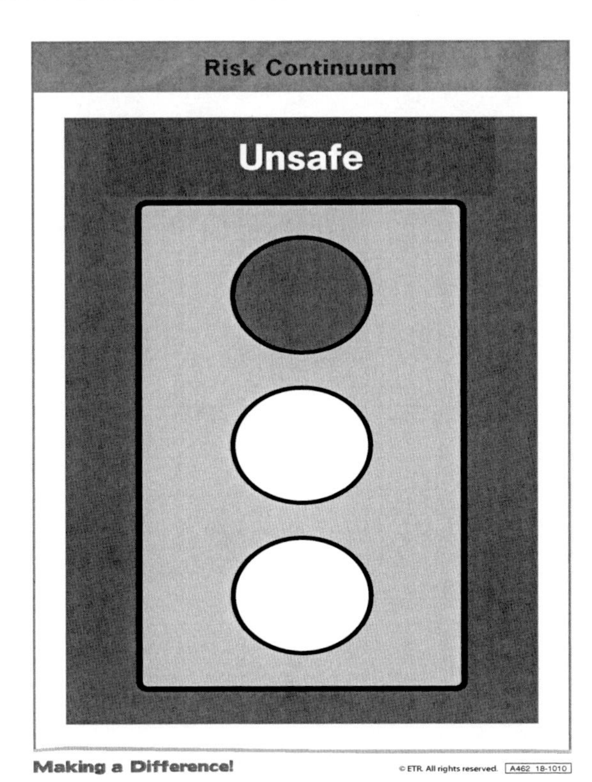

3 Posters

20 Cards

GIVING ADVICE ABOUT ABSTINENCE

GOALS

The goals of this module are to:

- Practice giving advice to their peers about the consequences of sex and the benefits of abstinence.

LEARNING OBJECTIVES

After completing this module, students will be able to:

- Explain information about HIV/STDs to their peers.
- Explain why abstinence is the safest and surest way to avoid pregnancy, HIV and other STDs.

MODULE PREVIEW

The fifth module: (1) Encourages students to think about their choices; and (2) provides opportunities for students to develop skills in giving correct information on HIV to friends.

STRATEGIES/METHODS

- Worksheet
- Information Hotline Exercise

MATERIALS NEEDED — INCLUDED IN IMPLEMENTATION KIT

- *Calling Koko Caller 1–3* handouts
- Blank newsprint

PREPARATION NEEDED

1. Be prepared to review key concepts from the fourth module.

INSTRUCTIONAL TIME: 45–60 minutes

ACTIVITY   MINUTES NEEDED

Pre-Activity: Key Concept Review   5
A. Nat Next Door 20–25
B. Calling Koko 20–30

 Making a Difference! For Youth with Cognitive Impairments

PREPARING FOR THE ACTIVITY

RATIONALE

Providing students with a brief review of key topics discussed in the previous module will reinforce their learning, prime them for new learning and help transition to the concepts in the upcoming module.

MATERIALS

None

TIME

5 minutes

PROCEDURE

1. **Begin by writing the names of key concepts learned in the last module on the board:**

   » HIV
   HIV, the virus that causes AIDS, damages the body's immune system. There is no cure for HIV, but there are treatments.

   » How people get HIV
   People can get HIV through unprotected sex or sharing needles. Some sexual behaviors, such as having sex with someone who is having sex with other people or having anal sex, have more risk of transmitting HIV than others, such as hugging, kissing, or holding hands. A person cannot get HIV through touching, hugging, coughing, sneezing, sharing food or utensils, insect bites or toilet seats.

   » How to prevent HIV
   Abstinence from sex and never sharing needles can prevent a person from getting HIV.

2. **Ask for a volunteer to explain what one of the concepts means.**

3. **Clarify concept if needed.**

4. Check for understanding with a few other students. Repeat process with the remaining concepts.

5. Tell students that last time the group learned how young people can protect themselves from the consequences of sex, including HIV. This time they will learn how to give advice about abstinence.

Making a Difference! For Youth with Cognitive Impairments

NAT NEXT DOOR

PREPARING FOR THE ACTIVITY

RATIONALE

This partially scripted roleplay activity provides an opportunity for students to be advocates for abstinence, further internalizing this option as the healthiest choice for people their age. Sometimes people (including adults) need to hear their own advice before the message is internalized.

ACTIVITY LEARNING OBJECTIVES

- Explain information about HIV/STDs to their peers.
- Explain why abstinence is the safest and surest way to avoid pregnancy, HIV and other STDs.

MATERIALS

None

TIME

20–25 minutes

PROCEDURE

1a. Introduce this activity by explaining that people often find it a lot easier to give advice to other people than to follow that same advice themselves.

1b. Tell students that as a group they're going to pretend that they have a neighbor who is thinking about having sex, and need to decide what advice to give to convince this person to remain abstinent.

FACILITATOR'S NOTE

You may want to prepare chart paper ahead of time with Nat's lines written out and blank space for the responses you generate with the class.

2.   Read the class the following introduction:

> You've lived next door to your good friend Nat for a long time. Nat is dating someone named Emery and you've seen them kissing. You know that Emery has had sex before. You're worried that Nat will decide to have sex with Emery and you think that Nat is too young.
>
> Nat comes over to talk and says, "Hey, Emery thinks we've been together long enough that we should have sex. I'm not sure about it. Can we talk?"

3.   Ask students for ideas for how to respond to Nat. Come to a consensus before moving on to Nat's next line.

4.   Repeat this process for the rest of Nat's lines:

> **Nat:** But I really care about Emery. I've never dated anyone before and I'm afraid Emery will find somebody else if we don't start having sex.
>
> **Class:**
>
> **Nat:** I'll have sex one day, so why not now? A lot of my friends are doing it. What's the harm?
>
> **Class:**
>
> **Nat:** I know Emery really cares about me and would never let something bad happen to me. We text each other all the time and Emery says I'm special.
>
> **Class:**

5.   Next, have the class generate ideas of what Nat decides to do and what Nat says next.

6.   Process this activity by asking the following questions:

> - Do you think you could convince a friend, brother, sister or cousin to wait to have sex with the advice you gave?
>
> - Why do you think it is important for young people to wait to have sex?
>
> - Would you follow this same advice if it was given to you? Why or why not?

B — CALLING KOKO

PREPARING FOR THE ACTIVITY

RATIONALE

Practice in advocating abstinence builds students' self-efficacy to safely resolve risky situations and practice abstinence in their own lives.

ACTIVITY LEARNING OBJECTIVES

- Explain information about HIV/STDs to their peers.
- Explain why abstinence is the safest and surest way to avoid pregnancy, HIV and other STDs.

MATERIALS

- *Calling Koko Caller 1–3* handouts
- Blank newsprint

TIME

20–30 minutes

PROCEDURE

1a. Tell students that in this activity they are going to practice giving more advice to people who have questions or concerns about abstinence and unintended pregnancy, HIV and other STDs.

1b. Explain that as a group they will take on the role of Koko, who has an HIV Information Hotline called *Calling Koko*.

2. Distribute the *Calling Koko* handouts.

FACILITATOR'S NOTE

If the handouts will detract from students' engagement, you may want to prepare chart paper or a slide deck with the Koko scenarios ahead of time.

3. Read aloud the first scenario, then brainstorm with the class advice to give to the caller. Encourage students to advise the caller to make a proud and responsible choice. Record main points on blank newsprint.

4. Using the following suggested responses, discuss any points that students do not come up with themselves.

FACILITATOR'S NOTE

Suggested responses are provided. Students' answers do not have to match the suggested responses word for word to be considered correct. However, in the large group discussion it is important to make sure that the points for each caller get discussed. You may want to read the suggested responses as a review before going on to the next caller.

5. Repeat steps 3 and 4 with the remaining two scenarios.

6. Summarize by complimenting the good advice the class generated about using abstinence as protection against unplanned pregnancy, HIV and other STDs. Emphasize that you hope everyone in the class makes the responsible choice to follow this advice if they are ever in similar situations.

Making a Difference! For Youth with Cognitive Impairments

MAIN POINTS TO COVER

The surest protection against HIV is abstinence.

Avoid any sexual behavior that involves the exchange of blood, semen, vaginal secretions or rectal fluids.

Don't share needles.

CALLER 1

Koko,

I've heard that young people can get HIV. I don't want to take any chances of getting HIV. What's the best way I can protect myself?

Suggested Response to Caller 1

The surest way to avoid HIV is to practice abstinence. That means not having vaginal, oral or anal sex. Every time a sexual behavior involves an exchange of body fluids, you take a chance of getting HIV.

You are also at risk if you share any kind of needle with anyone for any reason (whether it's for injecting drugs, tattooing or ear piercing).

The proud and responsible thing to do is to practice abstinence and not share needles.

MAIN POINTS TO COVER

Commitment in a relationship is not an effective form of protection.

Abstinence is the surest way to prevent HIV.

Talk it out.

You have plenty of time for sex when you're older.

CALLER 2

Dear Koko,

My friend and I really love each other, and we've been thinking about having sex, but only with each other. I trust my friend, but I'm concerned about HIV. We are both 14 years old, and we don't use drugs or share needles. Do we have to worry about HIV?

Suggested Response to Caller 2

If you and your friend have never had vaginal, oral or anal sex with anyone else or shared needles of any kind, the chances are that neither of you has HIV.

However, to avoid any possibility of future infection, I would suggest that you avoid vaginal, oral and anal sex. Deciding to have sex with someone is a big decision and it involves thinking about how you will protect yourselves from HIV, other STDs and unplanned pregnancy, if you are with someone of the opposite sex.

You'll have plenty of time for those things when you're older. Talk it over and decide together why it is best to wait right now. Even though you were thinking about having sex only with each other, that alone is not considered very good protection against HIV.

CALLER 3

Hi Koko,

I am 16 years old, and my girlfriend and I have never had vaginal sex. We do other things, though, including oral sex to make sure that she doesn't get pregnant. I hear that teens my age are getting sexually transmitted diseases. Is oral sex safe? How do we protect ourselves from STDs?

Suggested Response to Caller 3

ALL sexually transmitted diseases, including HIV, can be transmitted during oral sex. Practicing abstinence is the surest way that you and your girlfriend can avoid unplanned pregnancy and STDs. That means avoiding vaginal, oral and anal sex altogether.

This is your surest protection against unplanned pregnancy and STD infection. From what you've told me, you already know there are other things that people can do to show affection and feel good that will not lead to pregnancy or transmission of disease. It sounds like you have a good relationship. Talk it out with your girlfriend and agree to avoid any sexual behaviors that could cause pregnancy or transmit an STD.

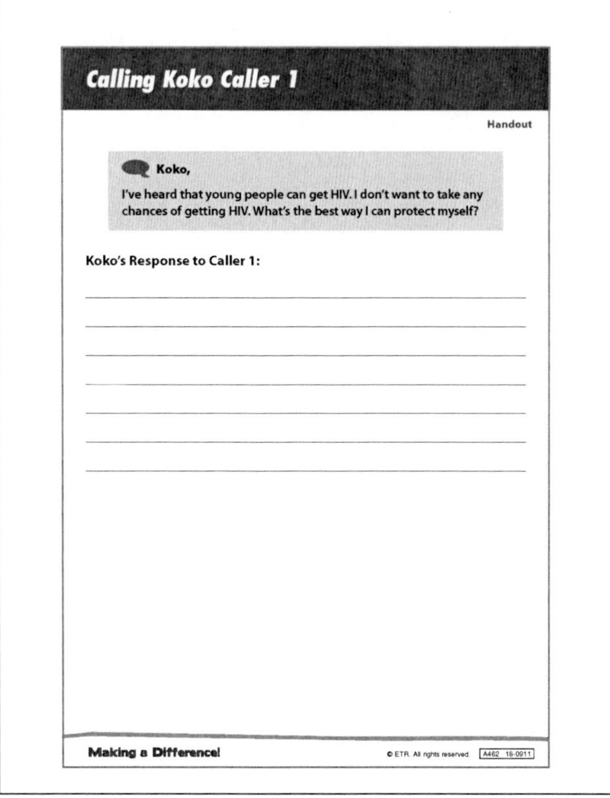

3 Handouts

Making a Difference! For Youth with Cognitive Impairments

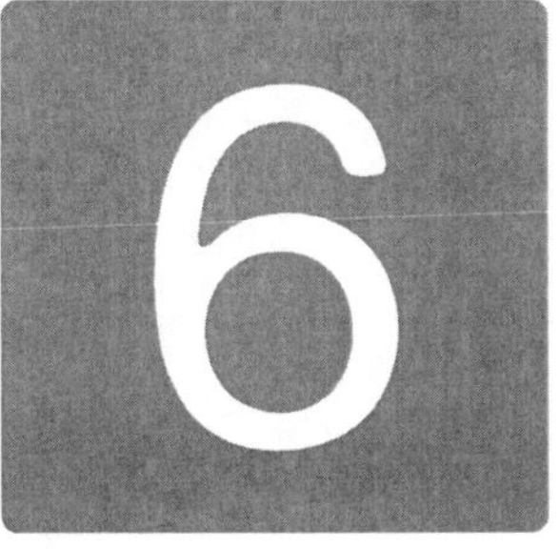

6

MODULE

ATTITUDES ABOUT ABSTINENCE AND USING PROBLEM SOLVING TO STAY ABSTINENT

GOALS

The goals of this module are to:

- Introduce students to problem-solving steps as a way of thinking through and coping with sexual choices.

LEARNING OBJECTIVES

After completing this module, students will be able to:

- Develop positive attitudes toward abstinence.
- State how using problem-solving steps can help avoid risky situations.
- State and explain the three steps of problem solving.

MODULE PREVIEW

The sixth module: (1) encourages students to think about their choices; and (2) provides them with a problem-solving strategy as a way to reduce their risk of HIV, other STDs and pregnancy.

STRATEGIES/METHODS

- Forced Choice
- Problem-Solving Strategies – Stop, Think and Act

MATERIALS NEEDED — INCLUDED IN IMPLEMENTATION KIT

- *Agree/Disagree* signs
- *Stop, Think and Act* poster

MATERIALS NEEDED — NOT INCLUDED IN IMPLEMENTATION KIT

- Masking tape

PREPARATION NEEDED

1. Hang the *Stop, Think and Act* poster.
2. Hang the *Agree/Disagree* signs.
3. Prepare to review and define the following terms (definitions in the glossary) throughout the lesson as needed:

   » decision

   » equality

   » open communication

   » respect

   » trust

4. Be prepared to review key concepts from the fifth module.

INSTRUCTIONAL TIME: 45–60 minutes

ACTIVITY	MINUTES NEEDED
Pre-Activity: Key Concept Review	5
A. Attitudes About Abstinence	15–20
B. Stop, Think and Act—Introduction to Problem Solving	10–15
C. Sean and Morgan Case Study: Problem Solving	15–20

 Making a Difference! For Youth with Cognitive Impairments

PREPARING FOR THE ACTIVITY

RATIONALE

Providing students with a brief review of key topics discussed in the previous module will reinforce their learning, prime them for new learning and help transition to the concepts in the upcoming module.

MATERIALS

None

TIME

5 minutes

PROCEDURE

1. Begin by writing the names of key concepts learned in the previous modules on the board:

   » Being Proud and Responsible
   Valuing yourself and making healthy choices, such as abstinence.

   » Abstinence
   Choosing not to do any sexual behaviors that could cause pregnancy or spread disease.

   » Self-esteem
   The way someone feels about themselves. Someone with high self-esteem won't let anything stand in the way of their goals, while someone with low self-esteem may allow themselves to be pressured into things they don't want to do such as having sex.

2. Ask for a volunteer to explain what one of the concepts means.

3. Clarify concept if needed.

4. Check for understanding with a few other students. Repeat process with the remaining concepts.

5.   Define any terms from this module that you expect your students will need to have defined before beginning the lesson. Terms may include:

   » decision

   » equality

   » open communication

   » respect

   » trust

6.   Tell students that last time the group learned how to give advice about abstinence. This time they will learn how to use problem solving as a way of thinking through and coping with sexual choices.

PREPARING FOR THE ACTIVITY

RATIONALE

Attitudes about abstinence affect the practice of abstinence. This activity strengthens positive attitudes toward abstinence and encourages students to question negative attitudes toward abstinence.

ACTIVITY LEARNING OBJECTIVE

- Develop positive attitudes toward abstinence.

MATERIALS

- Agree/Disagree signs

TIME

15–20 minutes

PROCEDURE

1. Tape the *Agree* and *Disagree* signs on opposite sides of the room.

FACILITATOR'S NOTE

If having students travel between the opposite sides of the classroom will not work for your class, you may choose to distribute "Agree/Disagree" signs for students to hold up their selection, or simply have students use the "thumbs up" symbol for agree and "thumbs down" for disagree.

2a. Introduce the activity by saying,

KEY MESSAGE:

Even if we have a lot of knowledge about sex, our attitudes and beliefs can get in the way of choosing abstinence.

> Having knowledge about sex is important. It's also important for us to think about our attitudes toward sex. Our attitudes and beliefs can lead us to do things even if we "know" we shouldn't.
>
> For example, a person may know having sex could interfere with their goals, but decide to have sex anyway because they believe their partner will break up with them if they don't.

2b. Explain that this next activity is a way to look more closely at attitudes about abstinence.

3. Explain that you are going to read some statements. Tell students they will then stand under the sign that best reflects their feelings about each statement. They are not allowed to stay in the middle, but must take a stand. If they agree with a statement, they stand under the Agree sign. If they disagree, they stand under the Disagree sign. Explain once they are in position, you will ask them to explain their choice.

FACILITATOR'S NOTE

If everyone stands under the same sign, ask students why they think no one chose the other option. If only one student stands under a sign, compliment this person for having the courage to make a choice that differs from the group and carefully ask why the student made that choice. Be sure the student clearly understood the statement. Give students a chance to change their minds after the explanations and before you move on to the next statement.

4. Read each of the following attitude statements.

 Making a Difference! For Youth with Cognitive Impairments

ATTITUDE STATEMENTS

- Guys who wait to have sex are "wimpy" or strange.
  (*Start with the agree side in the discussion.*)

- The more you like and respect yourself, the easier it is to abstain from sex.
  (*Start with the disagree side in the discussion.*)

- If someone didn't respect my decision to wait to have sex, I would find someone else who would respect my choice.

- People who wait to have sex are boring and unpopular.

- It is a female partner's responsibility to set sexual limits.

- There are other pleasurable sexual behaviors people can engage in besides sexual intercourse.

- It is harder for a male to say no to sex than it is for a female.

- Young people who choose to wait to have sex are proud and responsible and have goals and plans for their future.

4.   Summarize by saying,

KEY MESSAGE:

People have different opinions about abstinence.

The surest way to protect yourself from unplanned pregnancy and STDs is choosing to be abstinent.

This is a proud and responsible choice.

In this activity, you can see that people can have different attitudes and opinions about abstinence. It's important to know that attitudes and opinions can have a strong influence on decision making about sex. Good decisions are based on respecting and protecting yourself, understanding possible consequences, and being proud and responsible. For many young people, the best decision may be to abstain from sex so that it is easier to reach their goals. People can always make the choice to practice abstinence, even if they've had sex before.

STOP, THINK AND ACT— INTRODUCTION TO PROBLEM SOLVING

PREPARING FOR THE ACTIVITY

RATIONALE

By learning a problem-solving technique, students will have a strategy they can rely on when faced with sexual decisions, rather than relying on emotions.

ACTIVITY LEARNING OBJECTIVE

- State how using problem-solving steps can help avoid risky situations.

MATERIALS

- *Stop, Think and Act* poster
- Masking tape

TIME

10–15 minutes

PROCEDURE

1. Display the *Stop, Think and Act* poster.

2a. Introduce the activity by saying,

KEY MESSAGE:

It can be hard to make healthy choices under pressure.

Feeling pressure and conflict is normal. Every day, people have to make decisions about all kinds of things while they are experiencing pressure and conflict. Often there's not much time to think about what to do. Without a strategy or plan, the choices people make at these times may not be healthy ones.

2b. Tell students that they are going to learn a problem-solving model that will help them think about making decisions under pressure.

3. Read the steps out loud one at a time, pointing to the poster so students can read along.

4a. Tell students the first step is Stop. Ask them why someone might need to Stop if they are being pressured sexually.

4b. Let students provide a few answers.

   Answers may include:

   » You might be feeling afraid, confused, angry or upset.

4c. Then explain that Stopping is important because it gives you a chance to take a deep breath, calm down and collect yourself.

5a. Tell the class the second step is Think. Ask students what someone might need to think about when being pressured sexually.

5b. Allow students to respond, then explain that Thinking keeps you, not your emotions, in control of a situation so you don't overreact or underact. The important thing here is to calm down and think things through a bit before acting.

5c. Tell students some things they might want to think about include:

- **What is the problem?**
- **What am I being pressured to do?**
- **What am I feeling? What is the other person feeling?**
- **What are my choices?**
- **What do I want?**
- **How can I stay in control?**
- **What alternatives can I suggest?**
- **What are the possible consequences?**

6a. Explain that once you are calm and have thought things through a bit, the next step is to Act on a decision.

6b. Say,

KEY MESSAGE:
After thinking about your options, it's important to make a choice and act on it.

Evaluate the possible consequences and make the best choice. Try it out and see how well it works. If your solution does not work well enough, you can try another alternative, or ask for help. Sometimes after taking an action, you realize it wasn't the best choice for you and you would do it differently the next time. That's fine. It's just important to reflect on what happened so you can learn from your experiences.

7. Transition into the next activity by explaining that the group will now practice the Stop, Think and Act problem-solving steps.

SEAN AND MORGAN CASE STUDY: PROBLEM SOLVING USING STOP, THINK AND ACT

PREPARING FOR THE ACTIVITY

RATIONALE

Applying the problem-solving steps to a situation will enhance students' ability to use them.

ACTIVITY LEARNING OBJECTIVE

- State and explain the three steps of problem solving.

MATERIALS

- *Stop, Think and Act* poster

TIME

15–20 minutes

PROCEDURE

FACILITATOR'S NOTE

The case study has been written to be gender neutral. Sean and Morgan might be a boy and a girl, a girl and a boy, two boys, two girls, or transgender youth.

1. Begin this activity by explaining that when we are pressured sexually, we often feel confused or upset and may not think clearly about how to deal with a situation. Explain that the class is going to practice using Stop, Think and Act to help practice abstinence in these situations.

2. Read aloud the *Sean and Morgan* case study.

SEAN AND MORGAN CASE STUDY

Sean is 3 years younger than Morgan. They've been going out for a while. They both really like each other, and Sean feels more grown-up and popular when they're together.

Lately, Morgan's friends have been talking about sex a lot and keep asking if Morgan and Sean have "done it" yet. Morgan figures it's time and starts to pressure Sean to have sex.

When Morgan asks Sean about having sex, Sean feels unsure about what to say. Sean has thought about it a lot, and even though Sean thinks Morgan is sexy, Sean doesn't feel ready for sex yet. Sean wants to wait until after high school to have sex. Sean does not want to do anything that might get in the way of future goals like graduating. Sean is also afraid of getting an STD and doesn't want to take any risks.

However, Sean really wants to keep the relationship with Morgan. Sean would be very hurt if Morgan had sex with someone else.

Today Sean and Morgan are hanging out at Morgan's house alone. They're kissing on the couch and things are getting hot and heavy. What can Sean do to avoid having sex?

3. Tell students that now it's time to practice Stop, Think and Act. Process the story with students by going through the following questions:

   » **Stop**
   - What can Sean do to stop?
   - What can Sean do to stay calm?

   » **Think**
   - What is the problem? What is Sean being pressured to do?
   - What do you think Sean is feeling?
   - What does Sean think Morgan is feeling?
   - What are Sean's choices?
   - What does Sean really want to do?
   - What alternative can Sean suggest to Morgan?
   - What are the possible consequences?

Making a Difference! For Youth with Cognitive Impairments

» **Act**

- What do you think is Sean's best choice?

- How should Sean act on that choice?

4a. Ask students how the age difference between Morgan and Sean affects their relationship. Ask if they have trust, respect, equality and open communication.

4b. Make the point that pressuring someone to have sex is not showing respect, and that the relationship is probably not equal. Morgan is 3 years older and is likely to be a lot more mature and experienced than Sean. Morgan probably has more power and influence in the relationship, which could put a lot of pressure on Sean. In healthy relationships, both partners are equal. One does not have more power than the other.

FACILITATOR'S NOTE

If you have time following this activity, you may want to consider leading the "Healthy Relationships" activity in Appendix A to reinforce the characteristics of healthy relationships.

5. Summarize as follows,

KEY MESSAGE:

Sexual activity may lead to pregnancy or STDs and can interfere with your goals.

Stop, Think and Act can help you make healthy sexual decisions.

That's how Stop, Think and Act can be used to think through a problem.

You know that having sexual intercourse can lead to STD/HIV infection or pregnancy, which can get in the way of reaching your goals. Using Stop, Think and Act can help you quickly make healthy sexual decisions and keep you on the path to your goals. It can help you make a difference and choose to abstain from sex.

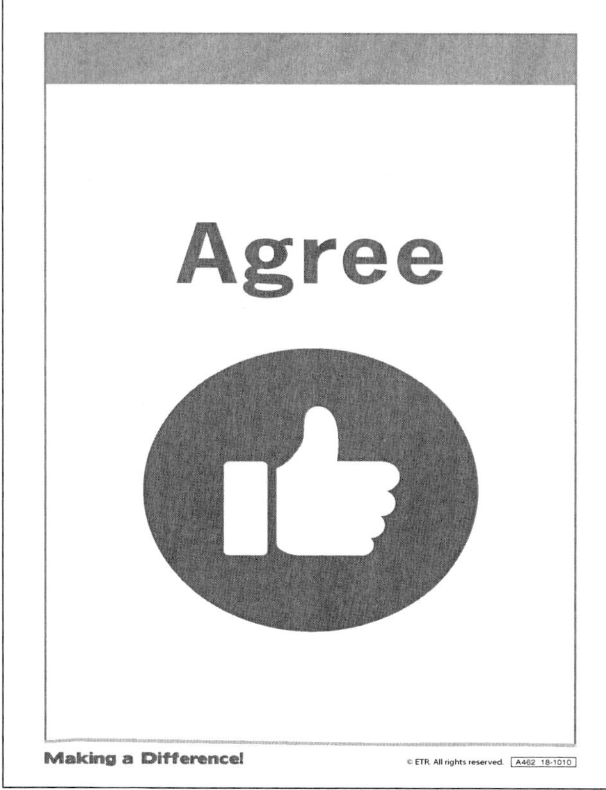

2 Posters

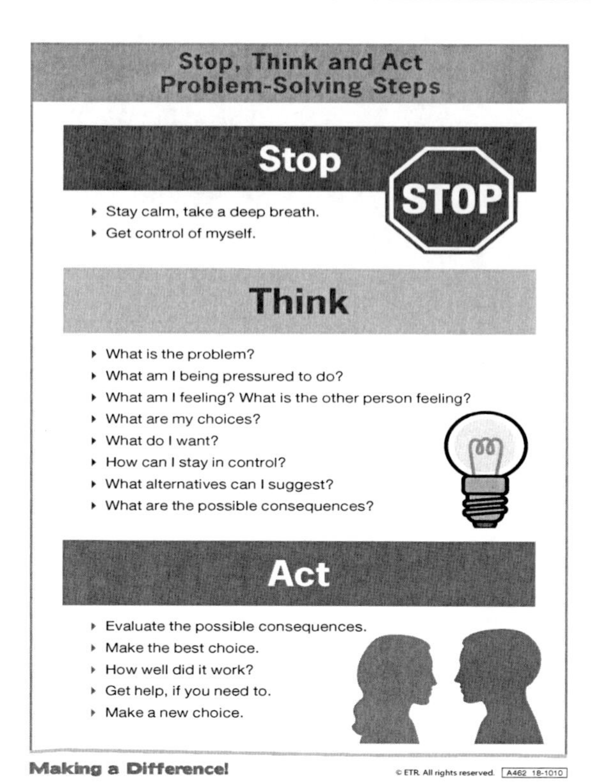

Poster

Making a Difference! For Youth with Cognitive Impairments

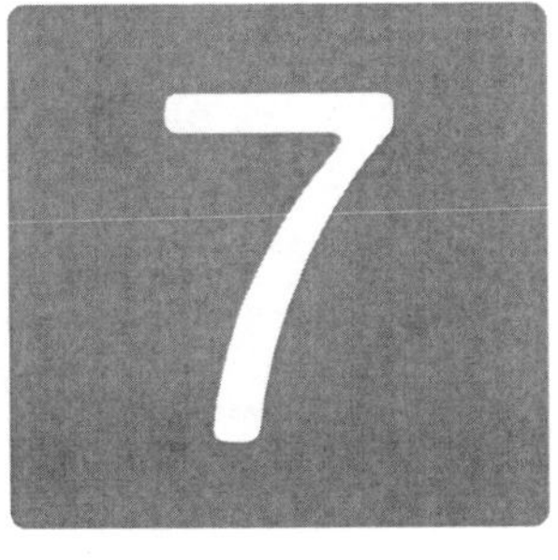

THE CONSEQUENCES OF SEX: STDS

GOALS

The goals of this module are to:

- Increase students' knowledge of sexually transmitted diseases.
- Increase students' perceived vulnerability to STDs.

LEARNING OBJECTIVES

After completing this module, students will be able to:

- Identify the signs and symptoms of the most common STDs.
- Identify how STDs, including HIV, are transmitted.
- Acknowledge their risk for contracting an STD.

MODULE PREVIEW

The seventh module: (1) helps students realize that they are vulnerable to HIV and other STDs; (2) helps them understand the importance of protecting themselves against HIV/STD infection by being abstinent; and (3) helps students identify their personal level of risk for HIV/STD infection.

STRATEGIES/METHODS

- Brainstorming
- Group Discussion
- The Transmission Game

MATERIALS NEEDED — INCLUDED IN IMPLEMENTATION KIT

- *STD* poster
- *Signs of STDs* poster

MATERIALS NEEDED — NOT INCLUDED IN IMPLEMENTATION KIT

- Pencils/pens
- Index cards for the Transmission Game—pre-labeled with Name and A, D or U
- Markers
- Newsprint
- Pre-labeled newsprint:
  - » *How STDs Are Transmitted*
  - » *Reasons to Avoid STDs*
- Masking tape

PREPARATION NEEDED

1. Label all of the newsprint charts as listed under Materials.

2. Hang the poster and pre-labeled newsprint charts in the order they will be used. Fold and tape the charts so the titles remain covered by the bottom half of the sheet until you use them.

3. Label the index cards for the game. On the back of the card write "Name: ________________". You may choose to include numbers 1-6 for each round of the game. On the front of the card mark A, D or U. Two students will have a "D" card, 6–7 will have an "A" card and the rest will have "U" cards. Increase the number of "A" and "U" cards in this approximate ratio for larger groups. An example card is pictured below.

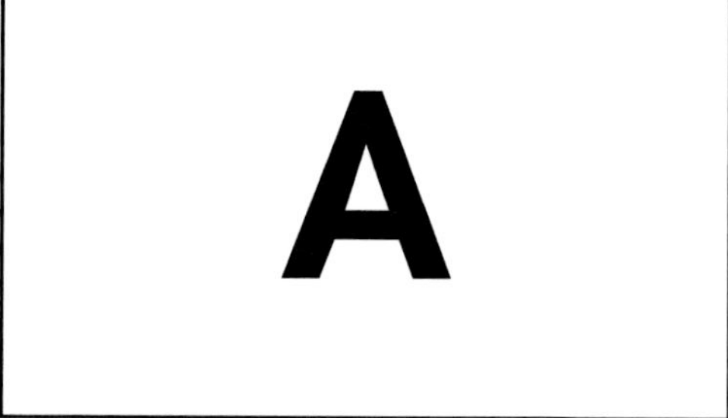

4. Prepare to review key concepts from the sixth module.

INSTRUCTIONAL TIME: 45–60 minutes

ACTIVITY	MINUTES NEEDED
Pre-Activity: Key Concept Review	5
A. Sexually Transmitted Diseases Brainstorm and Discussion	25–30
B. Don't Pass It Along: The Transmission Game	15–25

 Making a Difference! For Youth with Cognitive Impairments

PREPARING FOR THE ACTIVITY

RATIONALE

Providing students with a brief review of key topics discussed in the previous module will reinforce their learning, prime them for new learning and help transition to the concepts in the upcoming module.

MATERIALS

None

TIME

5 minutes

PROCEDURE

1. Begin by writing the names of key concepts learned in the last module on the board:

   » Stop, Think and Act
   A problem-solving model that helps youth make healthy decisions under pressure.

2. Ask for a volunteer to explain the concept.

3. Clarify concept if needed.

4. Check for understanding with a few other students.

5. Tell students that last time the group learned how to use problem solving as a way of thinking through and coping with sexual choices. This time they will learn the importance of protecting themselves against HIV/STD infection by being abstinent.

<table>
<tr><td>ACTIVITY
A</td><td># SEXUALLY TRANSMITTED DISEASES
BRAINSTORM AND DISCUSSION</td></tr>
</table>

PREPARING FOR THE ACTIVITY

RATIONALE

Providing information on STD transmission and symptoms gives students the information they need to prevent the spread of STDs. In addition, it provides a common ground for discussing attitudes and concerns about STDs and increases perceived vulnerability to infection as well as motivation to avoid infection through abstinence.

ACTIVITY LEARNING OBJECTIVES

- Identify the signs and symptoms of the most common STDs.
- Identify how STDs, including HIV, are transmitted.

MATERIALS

- Newsprint
- Markers
- *STD* poster
- *Signs of STDs* poster

- Pre-labeled newsprint:
    » *How STDs Are Transmitted*
    » *Reasons to Avoid STDs*

Reasons to Avoid STDs

How STDs Are Transmitted

TIME

25–30 minutes

PROCEDURE

1. Begin this activity by displaying the *STD* poster. Use newsprint to cover the poster so only the letters "S T D" are revealed.

2. Ask what the letters "STD" stand for.

    Answer:

    »   Sexually transmitted disease

3. Once students respond with the correct answer, ask students to brainstorm all of the STDs they know about or have heard of before.

4. **Uncover the poster and read any STDs they did not mention:**

» Chlamydia	» Herpes
» Gonorrhea	» HIV
» Syphilis	» HPV (human papillomavirus)
» Trichomoniasis	» Hepatitis B

FACILITATOR'S NOTE

If students use slang terms to name the STDs, determine what disease the person is describing (e.g., clap is slang for gonorrhea).

If students ask for more information about an STD, refer to the Supplemental Background Information on STDs in Appendix B.

5a. **Then explain that some STDs are curable and others are treatable:**

- **Curable**—These include chlamydia, gonorrhea, syphilis, trichomoniasis and pubic lice. You can take medicine that kills these STDs.

- **Treatable**—These include herpes, HIV, hepatitis B and HPV (human papillomavirus). These STDs are not curable. The symptoms can be treated, but the STD can stay in the body. Notice all the non-curable STDs start with the letter H.

6a. **Display the *Signs of STDs* poster. Read the list to students:**

- **Burning when peeing**

- **Sores, blisters, bumps, warts or pimples near the penis, vagina, mouth or anus.**

- **Unusual fluids from penis or vagina**

- **Rash or itch on or near the penis or vagina**

- **Frequent peeing**

- **Pain in the stomach area**

- **Often there are NO symptoms**

6b. Tell the group that if they notice anything unusual or not normal on their genitals, they should talk to a health care provider or their parent or guardian about it.

7. Then say,

KEY MESSAGE:

There are many different sexually transmitted diseases.

You may not be able to see when somebody has an STD, and they may not know they have one.

As you can see, there are a lot of different sexually transmitted diseases with a lot of different signs and symptoms. However, in many cases, a person can have an STD and have no symptoms! This means that people may not even know they have an STD. It also means that even if you don't notice any sores, blisters, warts or other signs, a potential partner still may have an STD.

8. Unfold the pre-labeled newsprint titled *How STDs Are Transmitted*. Ask the group how they think people get STDs.

9. List answers on the newsprint as the group responds.

Be sure the answers include:

» Vaginal sex (penis in vagina)

» Oral sex (a person's mouth on another person's penis or vagina)

» Anal sex (penis in anus)

» Mother to child (during pregnancy, at birth, or through breastfeeding)

» Sharing needles

» Skin-to-skin genital contact (herpes, syphilis, HPV)

10. Next ask who can get an STD.

Answer:

» Anyone who has unprotected sex.

Reiterate for students that unprotected sex is sex without a protective barrier (such as a condom).

Making a Difference! For Youth with Cognitive Impairments

11. Let students answer, and then say,

KEY MESSAGE:

Anybody can get an STD if they engage in unprotected sexual behaviors with a person who has an STD.

Young people are most likely to get an STD than any other age group. Abstinence is the only 100 percent sure way to protect yourself from STDs.

> That's right. Anyone who engages in unprotected sexual intercourse can get an STD. But teens and young adults are affected by STDs more than any other age group. The Centers for Disease Control and Prevention estimates that there are nearly 20 million new cases of STD each year, and that about half of these occur in young people ages 15 to 24.*
>
> The main way people get STDs is through sexual behaviors—oral, anal and vaginal sex. Some STDs (herpes, syphilis, HPV) can also be spread by skin-to-skin genital contact or touching. If you engage in any of these behaviors with a person who has an STD, you are at risk of catching it. Abstinence is the only 100 percent sure way to protect yourself from STD.
>
> *Centers for Disease Control and Prevention. 2014. Reported STDs in the United States. Available at: http://www.cdc.gov/std/stats13/std-trends-508.pdf. Accessed 9/13/18.

FACILITATOR'S NOTE

You may choose to look up and share local and/or state STD rates with students.

12. Now ask what is the one sure way to prevent getting STDs.

13. Let students answer the question. Then say the 100 percent sure way to prevent getting an STD is ABSTINENCE.

14a. Remind students that they now know how STDs are transmitted, the signs and symptoms that can indicate an STD infection, that some STDs don't have symptoms, and how to avoid getting an STD.

15. Unfold the newsprint titled *Reasons to Avoid STDs*. Ask students why they would want to avoid getting an STD, and have students brainstorm reasons. Suggest they think of some of the long-term physical and emotional consequences of getting an STD. List responses on the newsprint. Encourage all students to respond.

Answers should include:

- Higher chance of getting HIV
- Death (syphilis, AIDS)
- Cervical cancer (HPV)
- Genital warts (HPV)
- Infertility (gonorrhea, chlamydia)
- Child born with an STD
- Embarrassment
- Odor and discharge
- Loss of relationship

16. Explain that no one chooses to get an STD. Some people have gotten STDs from sex that was against their will. Summarize this activity by saying,

KEY MESSAGE:

Anyone can get an STD.

KEY MESSAGE:

STDs increase the chance of HIV infection.

KEY MESSAGE:

STDs can have serious emotional and physical consequences.

There are four important facts about STDs that I want to emphasize:

1. Anyone can get an STD. Young people ages 15–24 make up half of all new STD cases. You or a partner can have an STD and not know it. Many people with STDs have no symptoms.

2. STDs increase the chance of HIV infection. They sometimes cause blisters or sores on or around the genitals, which can become a point of entry for HIV during sex.

3. STDs can have serious emotional and physical consequences, including possible death in the case of AIDS and untreated syphilis. The consequences for women are especially harsh and include things such as pelvic inflammatory disease, ectopic pregnancy, cervical cancer, infertility, chronic pelvic pain, and possible transmission of the STD to her baby. If a person is concerned about having an STD, it is very important to go to a doctor or clinic to get tested and treated.

(continued)

 Making a Difference! For Youth with Cognitive Impairments

KEY MESSAGE:

Some STDs cannot be cured, but all STDs are preventable.

KEY MESSAGE:

The surest way to avoid STDs is to abstain from sexual activity.

4. Some STDs cannot be cured, including HIV, but all STDs are preventable. Abstinence—not having sex—is the surest way to prevent STD.

Remember how STDs are transmitted, what can happen if you get infected, reasons to avoid them and how to avoid them. The surest way to avoid STDs is to abstain from oral, anal and vaginal sex, and from any kind of skin-to-skin genital contact that can transmit them.

<table>
<tr><td>ACTIVITY
B</td><td>DON'T PASS IT ALONG:
THE TRANSMISSION GAME</td></tr>
</table>

PREPARING FOR THE ACTIVITY

RATIONALE

Participating in an exercise that highlights how easy it is to get an STD breaks down students' feelings of invulnerability and can increase their motivation to practice abstinence.

ACTIVITY LEARNING OBJECTIVE

- Acknowledge their risk for contracting an STD.

MATERIALS

- Lettered index cards (A, U, and D)
- Pencils/pens

TIME

15–25 minutes

PROCEDURE

1. Introduce the activity. Explain that the class is going to participate in an activity that will help them understand how people get STDs.

> ### FACILITATOR'S NOTE
>
> This activity illustrates how easy it is to transmit an STD if people have unprotected intercourse. This is a fun, engaging activity but it can also be sensitive. Some students may have already had an STD; some might be living with HIV; and others may have family members or friends who are affected by HIV. Make sure no one is stigmatized by the activity.

2. Distribute the lettered cards and pencils so that two students have a "D," six or seven students have an "A" and the rest get a "U." (Keep this approximate ratio if the group numbers are larger or smaller.) DO NOT tell students what the letters mean at this time.

A = Abstinence

U = Unprotected Sex (oral, anal or vaginal sex)

D = Disease (STD/HIV)

3a. Give the following instructions:

> • Listen carefully so you don't miss anything.
>
> • On the side of the index card that does not have a letter on it, write your name on the name line.
>
> • Walk around the class until I say "stop."
>
> • Pair off with the person standing closest to you.
>
> • I will read a question.
>
> • You and your partner will each answer the question and talk about your responses.
>
> • When I call time (about a minute), you will sign each other's card on the "name" side. Return the card to the original owner.
>
> • Then you'll move around the room again until I say "stop" and you will pair up with a new partner.
>
> • We will keep doing this until you've had six brief discussions.

3b. Model this process with a volunteer.

4. Begin the game. Read each of the following questions, following the procedure you just described. After each question, have students move to a new partner.

> 1. How would you feel if you got an STD?
>
> 2. Why is it a good idea for young people to wait to have sex?
>
> 3. What are some reasons young people give for wanting to wait to have sex?
>
> 4. When a couple doesn't have sex, what other things can they do together?
>
> 5. What would you think of someone who wanted to wait to have sex?
>
> 6. What might you say to someone who tries to talk you into having sex when you don't want to?

5.   When the six questions have been discussed, ask all students to have a seat.

6a. Explain that this has been an exercise involving "talking activity," but everyone should pretend that each conversation was an act of "sexual activity."

6b. Instruct everyone to look at their cards and tell them the letters on the cards represent something in this exercise.

6c. Ask the students with the "D" cards to stand. Tell them that for the purposes of this activity only, they have an STD and anyone whose name is on their card could have the STD too. Instruct them to read the names on the back of their cards.

6d. Instruct everyone whose name was read to stand.

7a. After the students whose names were called are standing, tell them if they have an "A" on their card it means they insisted on abstinence and refused to engage in sexual activity. Instruct those with "A"s to sit back down.

7b. Then explain that anyone who has a "U" on their card must remain standing because they took a chance and engaged in unprotected sexual activity and are now possibly infected with the STD.

8.   Ask the students still standing, one at a time, to read the names on their cards. Use the same process to find out the total number who got "infected" during this activity.

9.   Count the number of students standing and ask the group to consider what would happen if they each continued to have unprotected sex with new partners.

10. Ask standing students to sit down.

11. Ask the students with the "D" cards how it felt to imagine they had been infected with an STD.

12. Ask the students with the "U" cards how they felt about possibly being infected.

13. Ask the students with the "A" cards how they felt when they got to sit down because they had protected themselves by being abstinent.

Making a Difference! For Youth with Cognitive Impairments

14. Now ask what the class learned from this activity.

   Try to elicit the following answers:

   » One person can infect many by passing the disease to someone who passes it on to the next person.

   » STDs can be spread through unprotected vaginal, oral and anal sex, and sometimes through skin-to-skin genital contact.

   » People have sex, not only with their partners, but also with their partner's past sexual partners.

   » You can't tell just by looking at someone who is infected and who isn't.

   » Anyone can get an STD regardless of whether the sex was consensual or forced.

   » There are other things people can do besides vaginal, oral and anal sex to show they care about each other.

   » Practicing abstinence is the surest way to protect yourself from HIV and other STDs.

15. Emphasize the following,

KEY MESSAGE:

Infections spread easily. Abstinence protects you from STDs.

This was just a game. However, it does highlight how fast and easily an STD can spread. The surest way to avoid infection is to practice abstinence, which means choosing not to engage in vaginal, oral or anal intercourse, and to avoid skin-to-skin genital touching.

16. Take the cards back and formally remove the disease from the students with the "D" cards to avoid any future stigma. Call out the names of students with "D" cards and tell them you are taking the card and the disease away from them.

17. Summarize as follows,

KEY MESSAGE:

Unlike in this game, STDs are real, and abstinence is the only 100 percent sure way to protect yourself from them.

STD infections among young people are real. It's important to understand the importance of practicing abstinence in your relationships to keep yourself safe. Remember, abstinence is the only 100 percent sure way to keep from getting an STD.

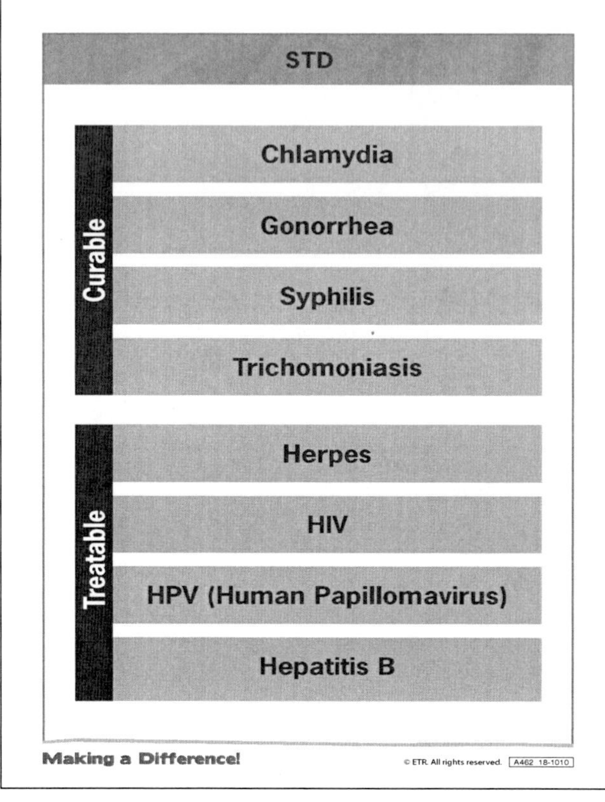

Poster

Poster

Making a Difference! For Youth with Cognitive Impairments

MODULE 8

THE CONSEQUENCES OF SEX: PREGNANCY: PART 1

GOALS

The goals of this module are to:

- Increase students' understanding of pregnancy as a consequence of sex.

- Increase students' perception that they are vulnerable to getting pregnant or getting someone pregnant.

- Increase students' understanding of the consequences of unplanned pregnancy.

LEARNING OBJECTIVES

After completing this module, students will be able to:

- Distinguish myths from facts about pregnancy.

- Express positive feelings toward pregnancy prevention.

MODULE PREVIEW

The eighth module: (1) helps students examine myths and facts about pregnancy; and (2) encourages students to abstain from behaviors that place them at risk for unintended pregnancy.

STRATEGIES/METHODS

- True or False Game
- Group Discussion
- Scripted Roleplay

MATERIALS NEEDED — INCLUDED IN IMPLEMENTATION KIT

- Pregnancy Statements: True or False (included in module)

- *Your Birthday Gift* handouts (3 copies, 1 for facilitator, 2 for student volunteers)

MATERIALS NEEDED — NOT INCLUDED IN IMPLEMENTATION KIT

None

PREPARATION NEEDED

1. Prepare to review and define the following terms (definitions in the glossary) throughout the lesson as needed:

   » dating

   » egg

   » ejaculation

   » menstrual cycle (period)

   » orgasm

   » pregnancy

   » roleplay

   » semen

2. Prepare to review key concepts from the seventh module.

INSTRUCTIONAL TIME: 45–60 minutes

ACTIVITY	MINUTES NEEDED
Pre-Activity: Key Concept Review	5
A. Pregnancy Statements: True or False	20–25
B. Your Birthday Gift (Scripted Roleplay)	20–30

 Making a Difference! For Youth with Cognitive Impairments

PREPARING FOR THE ACTIVITY

RATIONALE

Providing students with a brief review of key topics discussed in the previous module will reinforce their learning, prime them for new learning and help transition to the concepts in the upcoming module.

MATERIALS

None

TIME

5 minutes

PROCEDURE

1. Begin by writing the names of key concepts learned in the last module on the board:

    »   Signs of STDs
        Burning when peeing; sores, blisters, bumps, warts or pimples near the penis, vagina, mouth, or anus; unusual discharge from penis or vagina; rash or itching on or near the penis or vagina area; frequent peeing; pain in the stomach area. Sometimes there are NO symptoms.

    »   How people get STDs
        People can get an STD through: oral, anal, or vaginal sex; skin-to-skin genital contact; sharing needles.

    »   How to prevent STDs
        The 100 percent sure way of avoiding STDs is abstinence.

2. Ask for a volunteer to explain what one of the concepts means.

3. Clarify concept if needed.

4. Check for understanding with a few other students. Repeat process with the remaining concepts.

5. Define any terms from this module that you expect your students will need to have defined before beginning the lesson. Terms may include:

   » dating

   » egg

   » ejaculation

   » menstrual cycle (period)

   » orgasm

   » pregnancy

   » roleplay

   » semen

6. Tell students that last time the group learned the importance of protecting themselves against HIV and other STD infection by being abstinent. This time they will learn about pregnancy as a consequence of sex.

 Making a Difference! For Youth with Cognitive Impairments

PREPARING FOR THE ACTIVITY

RATIONALE

This activity helps students distinguish between myths and facts about pregnancy. Even if it is a subject with which they are quite familiar, they may continue to have misconceptions.

ACTIVITY LEARNING OBJECTIVE

- Distinguish myths from facts about pregnancy.

MATERIALS

- Pregnancy Statements: True or False (included in module)

TIME

20–25 minutes

PROCEDURE

1. Tell students you're going to play a game designed to help them learn some more about one of the consequences of sex—pregnancy.

2. Explain the directions to the room:

    - I'm going to read some statements about pregnancy.

    - After each statement, I want you to tell me if the statement is true or false.

    - I also want you to explain why it is true or false.

    - If you don't know, you can ask for help from your classmates.

3. Read the statements on the Pregnancy Statements: True or False page.

4. Supplement students' explanations with those provided after each statement or have other students give the information.

5. Once all the statements have been completed, compliment students on how they did and all the correct information they know.

6. Summarize by explaining that the more students know about the consequences of sex such as unplanned pregnancy, the better they will be at avoiding them. Tell them that next they are going to do some roleplays to help them practice saying no to risky sexual situations.

Making a Difference! For Youth with Cognitive Impairments

PREGNANCY STATEMENTS: TRUE OR FALSE

1. **People can get pregnant before they have their first period.**

   TRUE

   A person may begin releasing eggs before their first period so it is possible to get pregnant even if they haven't had a period yet.

2. **You can't get pregnant/get someone pregnant the first time you have sex.**

   FALSE

   Of course you can! It happens every day.

3. **You can get pregnant even if the penis is pulled out before ejaculation.**

   TRUE

   Sometimes a person will pull the penis out before ejaculation to avoid pregnancy. This doesn't work all the time because it's very difficult for many people, especially teens, to actually pull the penis out before they ejaculate (or come). And, sperm can come out of the penis before ejaculation.

4. **You can't get pregnant if you have sex standing up.**

   FALSE

   Sperm doesn't care what position you're in. Any time semen comes in contact with the vagina, you can get pregnant.

5. **You can't get pregnant unless you have an orgasm (come).**

   FALSE

   It doesn't matter if you enjoy the sex or you don't. You can get pregnant if you engage in penis-in-vagina intercourse without using protection.

9. **You can't get pregnant if you swallow semen.**

   TRUE

   The only way you can get pregnant is if sperm cells enter the vagina, usually during sexual intercourse, and fertilize an egg cell.

6. **If a person misses a period, they're definitely pregnant.**

   FALSE

   When people first start having periods they may have them at different times of the month or even skip a month from time to time. But if a person has had sexual intercourse and then misses a period, they could be pregnant. They should get tested right away, and see a doctor if the pregnancy test is positive.

7. **Gay and lesbian teens don't need to know how to avoid pregnancy.**

   FALSE

   For many different reasons, gay and lesbian teens sometimes engage in penis-in-vagina intercourse—and if they do, they could create a pregnancy. For example, a lesbian teen can get pregnant after having sex with a guy. A gay teen guy can get his partner pregnant if he has sex with a female.

8. **There's no safe time of the month to have sex and avoid pregnancy.**

   TRUE

   True. There is no absolutely safe time of the month when you can't get pregnant or get someone pregnant.

10. **Having anal instead of vaginal intercourse is a good strategy for preventing pregnancy.**

    FALSE

    This is not a wise pregnancy prevention strategy because if semen gets near the vagina, then a pregnancy could happen. Anal sex is also high risk for STDs because the lining of the anus is thin and lubricates less than the vagina, so it's easy for STDs to enter the body that way.

YOUR BIRTHDAY GIFT

PREPARING FOR THE ACTIVITY

RATIONALE

Analyzing effective ways of handling pressure from a romantic partner can strengthen students' ability to resist partner pressure.

ACTIVITY LEARNING OBJECTIVE

- Express positive feelings toward pregnancy prevention.

MATERIALS

- *Your Birthday Gift* handout (3 copies, 1 for facilitator, 2 for student volunteers)

TIME

20–30 minutes

PROCEDURE

1. Introduce this activity. Explain that sometimes when a couple is dating, they may not always agree on what sexual activity they are willing and not willing to do. Tell the class you're going to look at what can happen when two people have different feelings about what they want to do when they are dating.

2. Read "Setting the Stage," and then ask for two volunteers who are strong readers to read Person 1 and Person 2. Give them each a *Your Birthday Gift* handout.

FACILITATOR'S NOTE

If only one person volunteers, the facilitator can be Person 1 and have the volunteer be Person 2. If no one volunteers, don't push it and read both parts. But try to get students to read.

YOUR BIRTHDAY GIFT

Setting the Stage:

It's your birthday. You and your partner are going out to a movie and dinner. You know that at some point having sex will be discussed. Your partner is willing to use condoms, but you're just not ready for any of it. You decide to tell your partner that you want to wait to have sex.

Person 1: Happy birthday, Honey! Here is a little something I bought, though I was hoping to give you another gift that doesn't come from a store.

Person 2: Do you mean you were hoping we would have sex?

Person 1: Yes. You don't have to worry. I have condoms.

Person 2: No. You are moving way too fast for me.

Person 1: We've been dating for a while. I love you, and I'm ready.

Person 2: Well, I'm not. I love you but I'm not ready to have sex with you. I know you are the person that I want to be with, but I also know that I need you to be understanding and patient. I want to have sex only when I'm absolutely sure—when I'm not scared or in doubt. So, the answer is no.

Person 1: Well, I don't want to feel like I'm pressuring you to do something you don't want to. It's important that you're sure. So, I guess I'll wait until you are ready.

Person 2: Thanks, for understanding. I love you so much and I'm really glad that you are willing to hold on for a bit.

3.   Then ask the following questions:

- How did Person 2 handle the pressure to have sex from Person 1?

- Why was Person 1 unable to convince Person 2 to have sex?

- What messages did Person 2 give about what Person 2 wanted or did not want?

- What showed that they loved and respected themselves as well as each other?

4. Summarize by saying,

KEY MESSAGE:

It is possible to say no to sex, even to someone you care about.

Sexual activity may lead to pregnancy or STDs and can interfere with your goals.

The proud and responsible thing is to abstain from sex if you are not ready.

It is possible to find a gentle but firm way to say no, even to someone you care about a lot. It's especially important to be able to do this in romantic relationships. You may be tempted to give in to the pressure because you are afraid of losing the relationship. But saying yes to sexual intercourse when you are not ready is never a good idea, and could even end a relationship. Giving in to pressure to have unprotected sex can put you at risk of pregnancy, HIV or other STDs. The proud and responsible thing to do is to abstain from sex if you are not ready.

 Making a Difference! For Youth with Cognitive Impairments

Your Birthday Gift

Scripted Roleplay

Setting the Stage:

It's your birthday. You and your partner are going out to a movie and dinner. You know that at some point having sex will be discussed. Your partner is willing to use condoms, but you're just not ready for any of it. You decide to tell your partner that you want to wait to have sex.

Person 1: Happy birthday, Honey! Here is a little something I bought, though I was hoping to give you another gift that doesn't come from a store.

Person 2: Do you mean you were hoping we would have sex?

Person 1: Yes. You don't have to worry. I have condoms.

Person 2: No. You are moving way too fast for me.

Person 1: We've been dating for a while. I love you, and I'm ready.

Person 2: Well, I'm not. I love you but I'm not ready to have sex with you. I know you are the person that I want to be with, but I also know that I need you to be understanding and patient. I want to have sex only when I'm absolutely sure— when I'm not scared or in doubt. So, the answer is no.

Person 1: Well, I don't want to feel like I'm pressuring you to do something you don't want to. It's important that you're sure. So, I guess I'll wait until you are ready.

Person 2: Thanks, for understanding. I love you so much and I'm really glad that you are willing to hold on for a bit.

Making a Difference! A462 18-0911

Handout

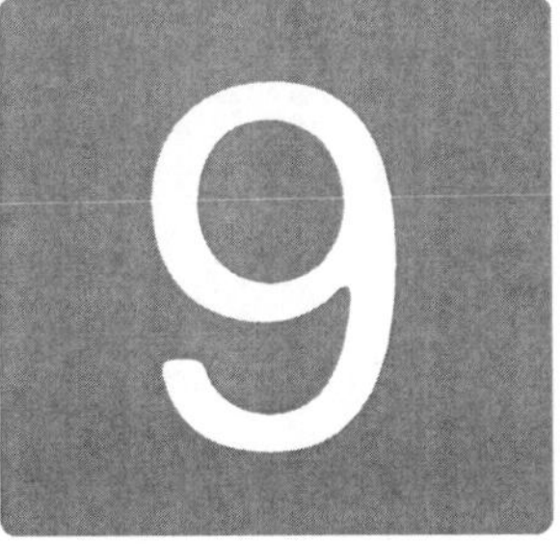# THE CONSEQUENCES OF SEX: PREGNANCY: PART 2

GOALS

The goals of this module are to:

- Increase students' understanding of pregnancy as a consequence of sex.

- Increase students' perception that they are vulnerable to getting pregnant or getting someone pregnant.

- Increase students' understanding of the consequences of unplanned pregnancy.

LEARNING OBJECTIVES

After completing this module, students will be able to:

- Express positive feelings toward pregnancy prevention.

- Identify negative consequences of teen pregnancy.

MODULE PREVIEW

The ninth module: (1) encourages students to abstain from behaviors that place them at risk for unintended pregnancy; and (2) illustrates how pregnancy can impact the lives of young people.

STRATEGIES/METHODS

- DVD Viewing
- Group Discussion
- Case Study

MATERIALS NEEDED — INCLUDED IN IMPLEMENTATION KIT

- *Jamal and Keisha* handout
- DVD: *Tanisha & Shay*

MATERIALS NEEDED — NOT INCLUDED IN IMPLEMENTATION KIT

- Pre-labeled newsprint:
  - » *Benefits of Waiting*
  - » *Delaying Strategies*
- Markers
- Masking tape
- Monitor and DVD player

PREPARATION NEEDED

1. Label all of the newsprint charts as listed under Materials.
2. Hang the pre-labeled newsprint charts in the order they will be used. Fold and tape the charts so the titles remain covered by the bottom half of the sheet until you use them.
3. Make sure the *Tanisha & Shay* DVD is set up and ready to play.
4. Prepare to review and define the following terms (definitions in the glossary) throughout the lesson as needed:
   - » birth control
   - » delay
   - » scholarship
5. Be prepared to review key concepts from the eighth module.

INSTRUCTIONAL TIME: 45–60 minutes

ACTIVITY	MINUTES NEEDED
Pre-Activity: Key Concept Review	5
A. *Tanisha & Shay* DVD	30–40
B. Jamal and Keisha—A Romance	10–15

 Making a Difference! For Youth with Cognitive Impairments

PREPARING FOR THE ACTIVITY

RATIONALE

Providing students with a brief review of key topics discussed in the previous module will reinforce their learning, prime them for new learning and help transition to the concepts in the upcoming module.

MATERIALS

None

TIME

5 minutes

PROCEDURE

1. Begin by writing the names of key concepts recently learned on the board:

    »   Consequences of Sex
        These could include sexually transmitted diseases (Module 7) or pregnancy (Module 8). These can make it harder for youth to achieve their goals.

    »   How to Avoid Consequences of Sex
        Abstinence, or not having sex, is the only 100 percent sure way to prevent or avoid pregnancy or STDs.

2. Ask for a volunteer to explain what one of the concepts means.

3. Clarify concept if needed.

4. Check for understanding with a few other students. Repeat process with the remaining concept.

5. Define any terms from this module that you expect your students will need to have defined before beginning the lesson. Terms may include:

>   » birth control

>   » delay

>   » scholarship

6. Tell students that last time they learned that pregnancy is a consequence of sex. This time they will learn how pregnancy can get in the way of achieving their goals.

 Making a Difference! For Youth with Cognitive Impairments

PREPARING FOR THE ACTIVITY

RATIONALE

Presenting and reinforcing information about pregnancy can promote further discussion. Seeing how pregnancy can impact the lives of individuals helps increase prevention planning.

ACTIVITY LEARNING OBJECTIVES

- Express positive feelings toward pregnancy prevention.
- Identify negative consequences of teen pregnancy.

MATERIALS

- Monitor and DVD player
- DVD: *Tanisha & Shay*

TIME

30–40 minutes

PROCEDURE

1. Tell students that the class is going to continue to focus on pregnancy prevention by watching a DVD called *Tanisha & Shay* in which sexually active teenagers deal with issues of pregnancy.

2. Show the DVD. Explain to students the DVD is divided into 3 parts. After each part you will ask the class some questions about what they just saw.

3. Show Part 1: Tanisha Finds Out. At the end of the segment, process by asking these questions:

- What did the medical provider tell Tanisha?

- What is your reaction? What do you think happens?

- Why do you think Tanisha and Shay didn't use birth control?

4. Show Part 2: Sharing the News. At the end of the segment, process by asking these questions:

> - How does the pregnancy affect everyone in Tanisha's life?
>
> - What does Tanisha risk losing because of the pregnancy?
>
> - What does Shay risk losing?
>
> - What did you think about Tanisha's mom's reaction to the pregnancy?

5. Show Part 3: Now What? At the end of the segment, process by asking these questions:

> - What did this video teach you about teen pregnancy?
>
> - Were these teens ready to become parents? Why or why not?
>
> - Tanisha's mom wants Tanisha to explore all her options. What are Tanisha's options?
>
> - How would your life change if you became pregnant or got somebody pregnant? How would you feel?
>
> - How would your parents react if you become pregnant or got somebody pregnant?

FACILITATOR'S NOTE

Be sure to understand current federal and state laws regarding adoption, abortion and safe surrender in order to provide accurate information to students.

Making a Difference! For Youth with Cognitive Impairments

6. Summarize this activity by saying,

KEY MESSAGE:

Pregnancy can change
your life.

Abstinence is the only
100 percent sure way
to avoid pregnancy.

Waiting to have sex is a
proud and responsible
choice.

As you can see, becoming pregnant or getting
someone pregnant can dramatically change your life.
Practicing abstinence is the safest and the only
100 percent sure way to avoid pregnancy.
Making healthy sexual decisions, including deciding
to be abstinent, is a proud and responsible choice.

ACTIVITY
B

JAMAL AND KEISHA—A ROMANCE

PREPARING FOR THE ACTIVITY

RATIONALE

This activity provides students with an opportunity to practice negotiation and refusal skills in preparation for real-life situations.

ACTIVITY LEARNING OBJECTIVES

- Express positive feelings toward pregnancy prevention.
- Identify negative consequences of teen pregnancy.

MATERIALS

- *Jamal and Keisha* handout
- Markers
- Masking tape
- Pre-labeled newsprint (folded so titles are covered; example on right):
  - » *Benefits of Waiting*
  - » *Delaying Strategies*

Benefits of Waiting

Delaying Strategies

TIME

10–15 minutes

PROCEDURE

1. Distribute the *Jamal and Keisha* handout. Ask students to follow along as you read.

FACILITATOR'S NOTE

You may choose to post the Jamal and Keisha story on a PowerPoint slide or pre-labeled newsprint if better suited than handouts for your class.

2. Read the story aloud:

JAMAL AND KEISHA

Keisha and Jamal are in the 9th grade. They've been going out for 3 months. They spend a lot of time together and love each other.

At first, they decided they didn't want to have sex. They thought they were too young. Keisha wants to save sex for marriage. So they haven't had sex yet, but they kiss and touch each other a lot.

Lately, Jamal's friends have been talking about having sex. This makes Jamal feel like he should have sex. He worries that he will be the only one among his friends who hasn't had sex yet.

Jamal is confused. He wants to respect Keisha's decision not to have sex but he doesn't want to wait until marriage. Jamal has started pressuring Keisha to have sex.

Keisha doesn't want to lose Jamal. Sometimes Keisha feels like she is the only one who isn't having sex, even though she knows that isn't true.

"Maybe sex isn't that special," she thinks. "But, then again, maybe it is." Keisha feels confused and doesn't know what to do.

One Saturday night, after a movie, Keisha and Jamal go back to Keisha's house to talk. When they get there, they find Keisha's mom has gone out and won't be back until much later. So, Keisha and Jamal are alone in the house.

3a. Process the story with the class. Ask the following questions, getting as many students as possible to share their answers:

- What are important reasons that Keisha might want to wait to have sex?

- What can Keisha say or do to delay having sex until she is ready?

- What are reasons Jamal would be better off waiting to have sex until he is older?

- What can Jamal do to help himself wait until Keisha is ready?

3b. Discuss the responses as needed.

4a. Unfold the pre-labeled newsprint titled *Benefits of Waiting*. Ask students:

- What are reasons that YOU might want to wait to have sex?

4b. Call on volunteers to answer the question. Record their answers on the newsprint.

5a. Unfold the pre-labeled newsprint titled *Delaying Strategies*. Ask students:

> • **What are things that you can say or do to delay having sex until you are ready?**

5b. Call on volunteers to answer the question. Record their answers on the newsprint.

6. Summarize this activity by saying,

KEY MESSAGE:

Making healthy sexual decisions can be hard, but it is the proud and responsible thing to do.

> Relationships can be complex. Making healthy sexual decisions in a relationship takes a lot of hard work, but it is the proud and responsible thing to do. We will be learning more about making those decisions and strategies to help you follow through on choices you make.

 Making a Difference! For Youth with Cognitive Impairments

Jamal and Keisha

Handout

Keisha and Jamal are in the 9th grade. They've been going out for 3 months. They spend a lot of time together and love each other.

At first, they decided they didn't want to have sex. They thought they were too young. Keisha wants to save sex for marriage. So they haven't had sex yet, but they kiss and touch each other a lot.

Lately, all of Jamal's friends have been talking about having sex. This makes Jamal feel like he should have sex. He worries that he will be the only one among his friends who hasn't had sex yet.

Jamal is confused. He wants to respect Keisha's decision not to have sex but he doesn't want to wait until marriage. Jamal has started pressuring Keisha to have sex.

Keisha doesn't want to lose Jamal. Sometimes Keisha feels like she is the only one who isn't having sex, even though she knows that isn't true.

"Maybe sex isn't all that special," she says to herself. "But, then again, maybe it is." Keisha feels confused and doesn't know what to do.

One Saturday night, after a movie, Keisha and Jamal go back to Keisha's house to talk. When they get there, they find Keisha's mom has gone out and won't be back until much later. So Keisha and Jamal are alone in the house.

Making a Difference!   © ETR. All rights reserved   A462 18-0911

Handout

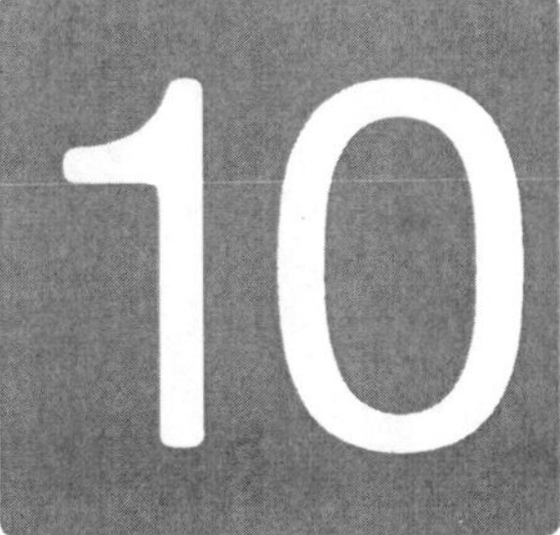

RESPONDING TO PEER PRESSURE AND PARTNER PRESSURE: PART 1

GOALS

The goals of this module are to:

- Increase students' awareness of the characteristics of peer pressure.
- Increase students' ability to resolve pressure situations.

LEARNING OBJECTIVES

After completing this module, students will be able to:

- Identify sexual messages from the media, peers and parents.
- Recognize pressure from peers to engage in sexual activity.
- Advocate for abstinence with other young people.

MODULE PREVIEW

The tenth module: (1) explores messages about sex that can contribute to sexual pressures; (2) provides students with practice in responding to peer pressure; and (3) helps students identify and practice refusal skills necessary to avoid a risky situation.

STRATEGIES/METHODS

- Group Discussion
- Problem-Solving Scenarios
- Forced Choice

MATERIALS NEEDED — INCLUDED IN IMPLEMENTATION KIT

- *Agree/Disagree* signs
- *Peer Pressure Scenario 1-4* handouts

MATERIALS NEEDED — NOT INCLUDED IN IMPLEMENTATION KIT

- Pencils/pens
- Masking tape
- Pre-labeled newsprint:
  - » *Delaying Strategies* (from Module 9—optional)

PREPARATION NEEDED

1. Hang the *Agree/Disagree* signs.
2. Be prepared to review key concepts from the ninth module.
3. Be prepared to review and define the following terms (definitions in the glossary) throughout the lesson as needed:
   - » peer
   - » pressure

INSTRUCTIONAL TIME: 45–60 minutes

ACTIVITY   MINUTES NEEDED

Pre-Activity: Key Concept Review 5
A. Understanding Messages About Sex 10–15
B. Understanding Peer Pressure 10–15
C. Responding to Peer Pressure 20–25

 Making a Difference! For Youth with Cognitive Impairments

PREPARING FOR THE ACTIVITY

RATIONALE

Providing students with a brief review of key topics discussed in the previous module will reinforce their learning, prime them for new learning and help transition to the concepts in the upcoming module.

MATERIALS

- Pre-labeled newsprint:
  - » *Delaying Strategies* (from Module 9—optional)

TIME

5 minutes

PROCEDURE

1.   Begin by writing the names of key concepts learned in the last module on the board:

     » Consequences of Sex: Pregnancy
       May make it harder for youth to reach their goals.

     » How to Avoid Consequences of Sex
       Abstinence, or not having sex, is the only 100 percent sure way to prevent or avoid pregnancy or STDs.

     » Delaying Strategies
       Things to say or do to delay having sex until one's ready. (Note: You can post the list of ideas youth already generated in Module 9.)

2.   Ask for a volunteer to explain what one of the concepts means.

3.   Clarify concept if needed.

4.   Check for understanding with a few other students. Repeat process with the remaining concepts.

5.   Define any terms from this module that you expect your students will need to have defined before beginning the lesson. Terms may include:

   » peer

   » pressure

6.   Tell students that last time they learned how pregnancy can make it harder to achieve their goals. This time they will learn about peer pressure and media influences that can make them feel pressured to have sex before they are ready.

Making a Difference! For Youth with Cognitive Impairments

UNDERSTANDING MESSAGES ABOUT SEX

PREPARING FOR THE ACTIVITY

RATIONALE

When students understand the sexual messages that stimulate their natural sexual curiosity, they will be better able to direct their curiosity appropriately.

ACTIVITY LEARNING OBJECTIVE

- Identify sexual messages from the media, peers and parents.

MATERIALS

None

TIME

10–15 minutes

PROCEDURE

1a. Begin this activity by explaining that one reason young people have sex is because they are curious. Tell students that sexual curiosity is normal, and increases as people get older.

1b. Explain there are sexual messages all around us that may increase young people's curiosity, and that they're going to look at some of these messages.

2. Ask students to name all the places they hear or learn about sex. There is no need to record the answers.

   Answers may include:

   - » School
   - » Friends/peers
   - » Parents/guardians/other trusted adults
   - » Religious groups or teachings
   - » Media (TV, movies, music, Internet, books and magazines, video games)

3. Ask students what their friends, partners or peers say about sex. There is no need to record the answers. Elicit as many responses as possible and encourage everyone to participate. Refer to the list below and add any messages that students did not mention.

Answers may include:

» Everyone is doing it.	» Nobody wants to be a virgin.
» Having sex makes you popular.	» You won't because you're scared.
» It feels good.	» Having sex makes you a man/woman.
» Trust me, I'll protect you.	» Wait until you're older.
» If you love me, you'll do it.	» You won't get pregnant.
» If you don't, someone else will.	» You have to if you're horny.

4. Ask students to think about the movies they see or the music they listen to. Ask what messages these things send about sex. Be sure to elicit specific messages, not just the name of the movie or song. There is no need to record the answers. Encourage everyone to participate. Refer to the below list and add any messages that students did not mention.

Answers may include:

» Sex is worth the risk.	» Dress, look, smell, act sexy.
» Sex is more important than feelings.	» People should show their bodies.
» No need to respect relationships.	» The more, the better.
» It's OK to have multiple partners.	» Casual sex is fun.
» No one else is a virgin.	» Everyone cheats in relationships.

5. Ask students how believing these messages might get in the way of achieving their goals. Encourage several students to give answers.

6. Ask what messages their parents or other trusted adults give about sex?

Answers may include:

» Don't have sex.

» Wait until you are married to have sex.

» Sex is not worth the consequences.

 Making a Difference! For Youth with Cognitive Impairments

7.   Ask students if anyone knows what "sexting" is.

Answer: When people send sexual messages and pictures using electronic devices such as cell phones, email and social networking sites.

8.   Ask students why they think people sext.

Answers may include:

- » They think it's fun and exciting.
- » It helps them feel attractive.
- » It's a way to initiate sex.
- » It's a way to show they're thinking about a partner.
- » They think it will get or help keep a partner interested.
- » A partner asks them to.
- » Their friends do it.

9.   Next explain reasons sexting is a bad idea:

- **You don't have control over what someone does with your pictures and messages. They could end up all over your school or all over the Internet.**
- **Sometimes people do mean things with the pictures and messages after a breakup and share it with their friends or online.**
- **If your pictures are put on the Internet it will be extraordinarily difficult to get them off.**
- **If your pictures are put on the Internet anyone can see them, including your family.**
- **There may be legal consequences. It is illegal to distribute a nude photo of a minor, even if that minor is you.**

10a. Ask students if they think it's safer if you don't show your face or crop your head out of pictures when sexting.

10b. Let students share their opinions, then explain that it's still pretty risky because pictures can be linked back to you through your email address, phone number, username, computer IP address or your relationship with the person you sent it to.

11. Then say,

KEY MESSAGE:

Sexting may seem fun, but it can harm your privacy, relationships and reputation.

> While sexting can seem like fun, you run the risk of other people seeing your very personal and private pictures and messages. It could hurt your reputation and relationships. There are plenty of other fun and safe ways to make your relationship exciting and keep you and your partner close.

12. Process this activity with the following questions:

> - Why do you think young people your age are curious about sex?
>
> - Do you think people your age are ready to handle the responsibilities and consequences of sex? Why or why not?
>
> - How do all of these messages affect you?

13. Summarize as follows,

KEY MESSAGE:

Sexual curiosity is natural and normal, but experimenting with sexual behaviors can have consequences, including pregnancy and STDs.

These can make it harder for you to reach your goals.

The proud and responsible thing to do is to wait to have sex to avoid the consequences of sex.

> Being curious about sex at your age is natural and normal. However, experimenting with sex to satisfy curiosity can be an unhealthy way for you to learn about sex. It can lead to the consequences we talked about earlier such as pregnancy and STDs, including HIV. These consequences can alter your life and get in the way of your goals. The surest way to avoid these risks is to practice abstinence!
>
> At your age, these are some proud and responsible things to remember:
>
> - It's OK to think about sex.
>
> - It's OK to talk about sex.
>
> - It's OK to develop feelings and attitudes about sex.
>
> But it's not a good idea to have sex until you are prepared to have sex with respect and responsibility. This is why abstinence is a good choice for you right now.

Making a Difference! For Youth with Cognitive Impairments

PREPARING FOR THE ACTIVITY

RATIONALE

If students understand how pressure from their peers can affect their sexual decision making and behaviors, even when the pressure is subtle, they will be better equipped to resist that pressure.

ACTIVITY LEARNING OBJECTIVE

- Recognize pressure from peers to engage in sexual activity.

MATERIALS

- *Agree/Disagree* signs
- Masking tape

TIME

10–15 minutes

PROCEDURE

1. Hang the *Agree* and *Disagree* signs on opposite sides of the room.

> **FACILITATOR'S NOTE**
>
> If having students travel between the opposite sides of the classroom will not work for your class, you may choose to distribute "Agree/Disagree" signs for students to hold up their selection, or simply have students use the "thumbs up" symbol for agree and "thumbs down" for disagree.

2. Explain that earlier the group talked about how peer pressure can influence young people's ability to make safe sexual choices. Tell students that this next activity will help them understand more about peer pressure.

3. Explain that you are going to read some statements. Tell students they will then stand under the sign that best reflects their feelings about each statement. They are not allowed to stay in the middle, but must take a stand. If they agree with a statement, they stand under the Agree sign. If they disagree, they stand under the Disagree sign. Explain that once they are in position, you will ask them to explain their choice.

FACILITATOR'S NOTE

If everyone stands under the same sign, ask students why they think no one chose the other option. If only one person stands under a sign, compliment this person for having the courage to make a choice that differs from the group and carefully ask why the person made that choice. Be sure the person clearly understood the statement. Give students a chance to change their minds after the explanations and before you move on to the next statement.

4. Read each of the following statements about peer pressure. As students explain their answers, reinforce all responses that show their understanding of peer pressure.

PEER PRESSURE AGREE/DISAGREE STATEMENTS

- It's hard to avoid having sex when all your friends are doing it.

- Young people who have sex are more popular.

- Girls don't pressure boys to have sex with them.

- Older guys pressure younger girls to have sexual intercourse.

- It is easy to say "NO" to sex when you are pressured by a partner.

- Most young people are having sexual intercourse, so it's OK to do it.

5a. Ask students to sit down. Once students have returned to their seats, ask what it felt like to be the only person under a sign. If it did not occur, ask them how it would have felt.

5b. Tell students that they have been participating in an activity on peer pressure. Ask what peer pressure is.

Answer:

» Peer pressure is when friends or other people around your age pressure you to do things you may not want to do. Or when you feel pressured to do something because people around you are doing it and you want to be like them.

  Making a Difference! For Youth with Cognitive Impairments

5c. **Ask what are some things friends or peers pressure each other to do.**

   Answers should include:
   - » Cut class
   - » Stay out late
   - » Smoke, drink alcohol, try drugs
   - » Have sex

5d. **Ask how peer pressure could have affected this activity.**

   Answer:
   - » Peer pressure could have affected whether people said they agreed or disagreed with a statement. If most of the other people agreed, a person might agree too, in spite of really feeling the opposite way.

6a. **Summarize by reminding students that of the many pressures on young people to have sex, one of the biggest pressures often comes from friends or peers.**

6b. **Explain that it takes hard work to resist peer pressure, but when they feel proud and responsible, they will make decisions for themselves and not just to follow peers. Explain that the group will now talk about how to resist pressure to have sex.**

PREPARING FOR THE ACTIVITY

RATIONALE

In this activity students consider how they would respond to peer pressure to have sex and have the opportunity to practice, in their own words, saying "NO" to sexual involvement.

ACTIVITY LEARNING OBJECTIVE

- Advocate for abstinence with other young people.

MATERIALS

- *Peer Pressure Scenario 1-4* handouts

TIME

20–25 minutes

PROCEDURE

1.   Continue the discussion about peer pressure. Remind students that one reason some young people have sex is because of peer pressure. Explain that they are going to discuss how to respond to pressure that comes from people close to their age. Tell them that, with the right skills, they won't have to give in to pressure to do something they don't want to do, such as have sex before they are ready.

2a. Ask students why they think a friend might pressure them to have sex before they are ready.

2b. Encourage several students to give a response to this question. Then say,

KEY MESSAGE:

Saying no to a friend can be hard, but you should do what you believe is right.

> It can be hard to say no to people you like. You may worry that a friend will get upset or reject you. You might feel left out, if you think that all your friends are doing something you're not. But sometimes you have to take a stand for what you believe is right.

3a. Continue by saying,

KEY MESSAGE:

Pressure to have sex often comes from romantic partners. If you don't know how to handle this pressure, you may go further sexually than you feel ready to.

> Even young people who don't have sex and have decided to be abstinent may feel pressured to say they do.
>
> Pressures to have sex often come from a romantic partner. Sometimes it's hard to know how to handle this pressure. Pressure can make people go further sexually than they want to, have sex when they're not ready, or lie about having sex when they haven't.

3b. Explain that now the class is going to look at some peer pressure situations and come up with ideas about how young people can handle these situations.

4a. Distribute the *Peer Pressure Scenario* handouts. Read each scenario aloud. After each scenario, go through the processing questions with the group.

FACILITATOR'S NOTE

Be sure to leave enough time to go through at least three of the scenarios with the group.

If the handouts will detract from students' engagement, you may want to prepare chart paper or a slide deck with the peer pressure scenarios ahead of time.

5. As students answer processing questions, support the following ideas as they come up:

> » Most people want to be popular, so it can be hard to do or say things that peers might make fun of or disagree with.

» It's important to make safe and responsible choices that are right for you, no matter what others are doing or want you to do.

» True friends will respect you and your choices.

» People who pressure others are not being respectful. It is disrespectful to pressure someone.

6. Compliment students on their ideas for how young people can deal with peer pressure. Acknowledge that there are lots of great reasons why young people choose not to engage in risky sexual behavior. Tell them that the more they practice responding to pressure, the better they'll be able to handle it. Remind them that they don't have the right to pressure anyone either.

FACILITATOR'S NOTE

Sample replies are given for some of the questions following the scenarios. Before you do this activity with the group, you may want to think about some possible answers to the questions that are not answered in case students need help.

SCENARIO 1

Jerome is talking with his friends. One of his friends keeps talking about the person he likes. Jerome thinks to himself, "I've never thought about someone that much. I'm so busy with school right now that if I got involved with someone, it might mess up my plans for the future." Then one of Jerome's friends asks, "How come you never talk about who you like, Jerome? What's the matter with you anyway?"

Jerome says, "Being in a relationship isn't the most important thing to me right now. I've got school and other things going on. I don't have a lot of time to spend with someone."

(continued)

 Making a Difference! For Youth with Cognitive Impairments

QUESTIONS FOR DISCUSSION

- What are some other things Jerome could have said? *("I have my future to think about." "Relationships can come later when I am ready.")*

- How is this peer pressure? *(Jerome's friends are pressuring him to talk or think about being involved with someone when he isn't ready.)*

- How important is it for young people to have their own beliefs and stick to them? Explain.

- How does it make you feel to be made fun of or questioned by your peers when you don't go along with the crowd?

SCENARIO 2

Alicia is at the movies with J.D., someone she likes from her class. While they are watching the movie, J.D. tries to hug and kiss Alicia. Alicia does not feel ready to hug or kiss yet and pushes J.D. away. Later J.D. says, "What's the matter with you? All those other couples are doing it." Alicia replies, "I just don't want to do that."

QUESTIONS FOR DISCUSSION

- What are some other things Alicia could have said? *("I wanted to watch the movie." "I guess I'm not like everyone else.")*

- Why might Alicia find it hard to say no if she really likes J.D.? *(She might worry that J.D. would spread a rumor about her or ridicule or reject her.)*

- Why should J.D. not pressure Alicia to go further than she wants? *(Because J.D. doesn't really know her yet. If J.D. really cares about Alicia, J.D. will respect her wishes.)*

- What do you think about giving in and doing something you don't want to do because of pressure?

(continued)

(continued)

SCENARIO 3

After school, Kenya invites Sammy and all their friends over because no one else is home. Sammy doesn't want to go because there might be pressure to kiss or do things Sammy doesn't want to do. Kenya says to Sammy, "Oh come on. All the popular kids are coming, and everybody else is having sex." Sammy says, "I don't care who else is coming, I'm not. Besides, I know a lot of our friends aren't having sex either."

QUESTIONS FOR DISCUSSION

- What are some other things Sammy could have said? *("I've decided to wait until the time is right and the time isn't right yet.")*

- What could happen if Sammy doesn't go? *(Sammy won't be pressured to do things Sammy doesn't want to do. Sammy can feel good about making a safe choice. Kenya might feel upset with Sammy, and not want to be friends anymore.)*

- What could happen if Sammy does go? *(Sammy might feel uncomfortable. Kenya might continue to pressure Sammy to do other things. Sammy could give in to pressure to have sex.)*

- How important is being popular if it gets in the way of achieving your goals in life?

- What do you think about giving in to pressure to have sex, even if you don't want to?

- -

SCENARIO 4

Ari and Drew have been going out for a few weeks. Ari wants to have sex, but Drew does not feel ready yet. Ari says, "You really turn me on. Come on, why don't we go somewhere where we can be alone?" When Drew says, "No," Ari says, "Why not? Don't you like me?" Drew says, "I'm just not interested in getting more involved right now."

QUESTIONS FOR DISCUSSION

- What are some other things Drew could have said? *("I don't think we want the same things." "I like you, but I don't want to have sex with you.")*

- How could Drew's decision affect the relationship? *(Ari could respect Drew's decision and they could grow closer. They might break up if Ari could not accept Drew's decision.)*

(continued)

 Making a Difference! For Youth with Cognitive Impairments

- What can Drew do to show Ari that their relationship is important without having sex? *(Talk about the decision, hold hands, hug, kiss, cuddle together, do fun activities together or with a group of friends.)*

- Is it OK for people to choose to wait to have sex when they are teens or young adults?

- What are some of the reasons Drew may have chosen not to have sex?

- Why can it be hard to say no in sexual situations?

FACILITATOR'S NOTE

If you have time following this activity, you may want to consider leading or revisiting the "Healthy Relationships" activity in Appendix A to reinforce the characteristics of healthy relationships.

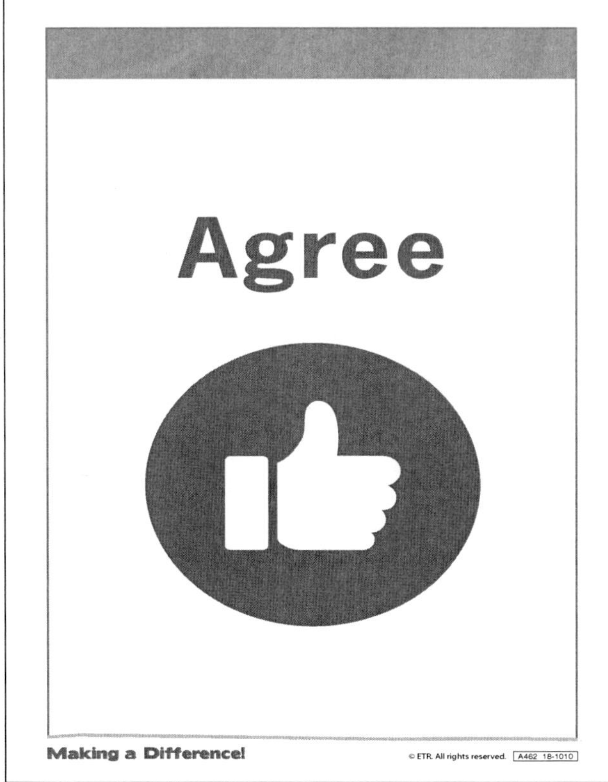

2 Posters

Peer Pressure — Scenario 1

Handout

Jerome is talking with his friends. One of his friends keeps talking about the person he likes. Jerome thinks to himself, "I've never thought about someone that much. I'm so busy with school right now that if I got involved with someone, it might mess up my plans for the future." Then one of Jerome's friends asks, "How come you never talk about who you like, Jerome? What's the matter with you anyway?"

Jerome says, "Being in a relationship isn't the most important thing to me right now. I've got school and other things going on. I don't have a lot of time to spend with someone."

Questions for Discussion

What are some other things Jerome could have said?

____

____

How is this peer pressure?

____

____

How important is it for teens to have their own beliefs and stick to them? Explain.

____

____

How does it make you feel to be made fun of or questioned by your peers when you don't go along with the crowd?

____

____

Making a Difference!   © ETR. All rights reserved.   A462 18-0911

4 Handouts

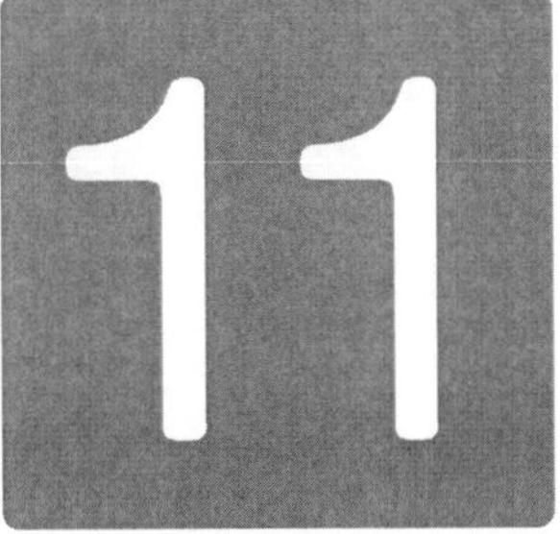

RESPONDING TO PEER PRESSURE AND PARTNER PRESSURE: PART 2

GOALS

The goals of this module are to:

- Increase students' ability to resolve pressure situations.
- Help students identify personal limitations and boundaries regarding sexual physical contact.
- Increase students' refusal and negotiation skills regarding abstinence.

LEARNING OBJECTIVES

After completing this module, students will be able to:

- Identify the specific sexual behaviors that fit within their personal comfort zone.
- Recognize pressure from peers to engage in sexual activity.

MODULE PREVIEW

The eleventh module: (1) provides students with practice in responding to peer pressure; and (2) helps students identify and practice refusal skills necessary to avoid a risky situation.

STRATEGIES/METHODS

- Problem-Solving Scenarios
- Roleplays

MATERIALS NEEDED — INCLUDED IN IMPLEMENTATION KIT

- *Showing Physical Affection* signs
- *Consent* poster
- *Refuse* poster
- *How to Say "NO"* poster
- *Examples of a Strong "NO"* poster
- Handouts:
    - » *While They're Out* (Scripted Roleplay)
    - » *While They're Out* (Unscripted Roleplay)

MATERIALS NEEDED — NOT INCLUDED IN IMPLEMENTATION KIT

- Markers
- Masking tape
- Blank newsprint

PREPARATION NEEDED

1. Hang the *Showing Physical Affection* signs.
2. Hang the *Refuse* poster, *How to Say "NO"* poster, and *Examples of a Strong "NO"* poster.
3. Hang the *Consent* poster and cover the definitions with blank newsprint.
4. Be prepared to review and define the following terms (definitions in the glossary) throughout the lesson as needed:
    - » boundary
    - » consent
    - » limit
    - » permission
    - » roleplay
5. Be prepared to review concepts from the tenth module.

INSTRUCTIONAL TIME: 45–60 minutes

<table>
<tr><th>ACTIVITY</th><th>MINUTES NEEDED</th></tr>
<tr><td>Pre-Activity: Key Concept Review</td><td>5</td></tr>
<tr><td>A. Knowing and Setting Physical Limits</td><td>10–15</td></tr>
<tr><td>B. Understanding Consent</td><td>10–15</td></tr>
<tr><td>C. Introduction to Refusals and Scripted Roleplays</td><td>20–25</td></tr>
</table>

 Making a Difference! For Youth with Cognitive Impairments

PREPARING FOR THE ACTIVITY

RATIONALE

Providing students with a brief review of key topics discussed in the previous module will reinforce their learning, prime them for new learning and help transition to the concepts in the upcoming module.

MATERIALS

None

TIME

5 minutes

PROCEDURE

1. Begin by writing the names of key concepts previously learned on the board:

    » Peer Pressure
      When friends or other people around your age pressure you to do things you may not want to do. Or, when you want to do things others are doing in order to fit in.

    » What happens when people give in to peer pressure about sex
      Peer pressure can make people go further sexually than they want to, have sex when they're not ready, or lie about having sex when they haven't.

    » How people express their sexual feelings
      Ways people express their sexual feelings to themselves or other people can include sexual touches such as kissing and vaginal, oral and anal sex.

2. Ask for a volunteer to explain what one of the concepts means.

3. Clarify concept if needed.

4. Check for understanding with a few other students. Repeat process with the remaining concepts.

5. Define any terms from this module that you expect your students will need to have defined before beginning the lesson. Terms may include:

   » boundary

   » consent

   » limit

   » permission

   » roleplay

6. Tell students that last time they learned about and practiced ways to resist peer pressure. Tell them in this session they will continue to practice resisting peer pressure and learn how to say "No" to sexual activity they are not ready for.

 Making a Difference! For Youth with Cognitive Impairments

KNOWING AND SETTING PHYSICAL LIMITS

PREPARING FOR THE ACTIVITY

RATIONALE

This activity provides students with an opportunity to practice negotiation and refusal skills in preparation for real-life situations. It is designed to help students determine comfortable limits for physically expressing affection and to explore ways of showing affection that do not involve vaginal, oral or anal sex, or any genital touching that could spread an STD.

ACTIVITY LEARNING OBJECTIVE

- Identify the specific sexual behaviors that fit within their personal comfort zone.

MATERIALS

- *Showing Physical Affection* signs
- Masking tape

TIME

10–15 minutes

PROCEDURE

1. Post the eight *Showing Physical Affection* signs. Spread the signs out around the room from left to right in the order indicated below:

    1. Give friendly looks and smiles
    2. Talk to each other
    3. Hold hands
    4. Put arms around each other

    5. Hug and kiss
    6. Touch above the waist
    7. Touch below the waist
    8. Have sexual intercourse

2a. Explain that these signs represent different ways of showing physical affection. Read the signs aloud.

2b. Instruct students to think about how far they think young people their age should go when showing physical affection.

3. After a few moments, have all of the students stand and move to the sign that matches how far they think young people should go when expressing physical affection.

4. While standing by their chosen sign, have each student answer why they chose that behavior as a stopping point or limit.

5. Bring students back to their seats and ask them to name some nonphysical ways to express love and affection.

    Answers could include:

    »   Write a love letter

    »   Give or make someone a gift

    »   Go somewhere fun together

    »   Put together a meal for someone

    »   Do something the other person likes to do

6. Support and encourage all reasonable answers. Summarize this activity by saying,

KEY MESSAGE:

Resisting sexual pressure can be hard, but it is the proud and responsible thing to do.

Talk with your partner ahead of time about what you are and aren't OK with doing. Be prepared to leave if you are pressured to do something you don't want to do.

Be proud and be responsible when dealing with pressure from other people. Knowing your own limits can help you do this. Try to avoid situations where you will have to stop someone from going too far. Talk about your feelings and what seems right for you in advance. If you and your partner can't agree, be prepared to leave. You may need to find someone else whose beliefs are closer to your own.

Making a Difference! For Youth with Cognitive Impairments

Module 11 // RESPONDING TO PEER PRESSURE AND PARTNER PRESSURE: PART 2

UNDERSTANDING CONSENT

PREPARING FOR THE ACTIVITY

RATIONALE

In this activity, students are introduced to consent. The concept is defined and explored through scenarios where students identify whether or not consent is present. This establishes how the negotiation of sexual behaviors should go, and lays the groundwork for the need for refusal skills when this negotiation goes awry.

MATERIALS

- *Consent* poster

TIME

10–15 minutes

PROCEDURE

FACILITATOR'S NOTE

Consent is an important, sensitive and highly nuanced concept. While this activity introduces the concept to support students' sexual agency before they learn refusal skills, it is beneficial to students if this topic is thoroughly explored and incorporated into their sexual health curricula. ETR's *Teaching Affirmative Consent* publication is a resource for facilitators on how to teach this topic, and includes an in-depth stand-alone lesson for students.

1. Begin the activity by asking students if they know what the word *permission* means. Affirm students' answers, and explain that asking permission is asking if you can or cannot do something.

2. Ask students what types of things they need to ask permission for.

   Answers may include:

   » Sitting next to someone

   » Borrowing something from a friend

- » Hanging out at a friend's house
- » Hugging
- » Holding hands
- » Going on a date
- » Kissing

3. Tell students that when people engage in sexual behaviors such as hugging, kissing or having sex, they need to get and give a special type of permission called *consent*.

4. Uncover or display the *Consent* poster. Tell students that consent means that both people clearly and freely agree to engage in sexual or romantic activity, and explain the rules of consent:

RULES OF CONSENT

- Both people must be awake, aware and able to make decisions.
  - **Example:** A person who falls asleep while kissing is not giving consent.

- Consent can be given with a person's words or actions.
  - **Example:** A person who says No, seems unsure, or seems upset is not giving consent.

- Consent for one thing or activity doesn't mean consent for another.
  - **Example:** If a person says OK to kissing, it does not mean they are OK with touching above the waist.

- People can change their minds at any time and can take back consent if they want.
  - **Example:** A person who said OK to holding hands can say they want to stop or that they don't want to hold hands again.

- Consent must be free from pressure, tricks, bribes or threats.
  - **Example:** If a person says that a friend has to hug them or they won't talk to that friend anymore, they are using a threat and are not following the rules of consent.

FACILITATOR'S NOTE

States, schools and other institutions may have their own definitions of consent that include additional points or otherwise vary from this definition. Be sure to check relevant policies and laws for your setting and adapt this definition to them as necessary.

5.   Clarify what consent is by asking the following questions:

- If someone is asleep, can they consent to sexual activity? *(No, they must be awake)*

- If someone is drunk, can they consent? *(No, they must be able to make decisions)*

- What if someone is confused or doesn't understand what's happening? *(No, they must be aware and able to make decisions)*

- If someone hasn't said No to sexual activity, does that mean they consent? *(No, the absence of a "no" does not mean "yes")*

- What if someone is being pressured or feels threatened in some way? *(No, consent must be free from pressure or threats)*

6.   Explain to students that there is one other important rule about consent. Tell students that people who are parents, family members or helpers (such as teachers, coaches, faith leaders, bus drivers and doctors) are not allowed to have romantic or sexual relationships with young people, and can never get consent for sexual behaviors from the people they are helping or are family members with. Even if a young person says "yes" and gives consent, this is never allowed.

7.   Tell students that now they are going to play Thumbs Up/Thumbs Down. Explain that you are going to read some stories. If the person in the story gives consent to sexual touches or actions, students should put their thumbs up. If the person in the story does not give consent, they should put their thumbs down.

- **Story 1:** Pat asked to kiss Jordan. Jordan said yes. Was there consent? How do we know?
    - *Answer:* **Thumbs up.** There was consent because Pat asked for consent out loud with no pressure, tricks or bribes and Jordan clearly said yes.

- **Story 2:** Jela told Casey that if they didn't kiss, Jela would break up with Casey. Casey then gave Jela a kiss even though Casey didn't really want to. Was there consent? How do we know?
    - **Thumbs down.** Jela broke the rules and used pressure and a threat to get Casey to give a kiss. Even though Casey kissed Jela, it was only because of the pressure. This is not consent.

(continued)

 Making a Difference! For Youth with Cognitive Impairments

- **Story 3:** Cam's bus driver offered Cam a kiss. Cam said, "No way." Did the bus driver follow the rules of consent?

  - **Thumbs down.** Helpers, like bus drivers, teachers or doctors, are not allowed to have romantic or sexual relationships with the people they are helping. Even if Cam said yes, the bus driver would still not have consent because of this rule.

- **Story 4:** Jessie asked Sam to snuggle while they were watching a movie. Sam said, "I'm not into snuggling right now, but could we hold hands?" Jessie said, "Yeah, sure." Did Jessie follow the rules of consent?

  - **Thumbs up.** Jessie did not pressure, trick or bribe Sam. Jessie respected Sam's wishes, and accepted the different activity Sam suggested.

8. Praise students for doing a good job figuring out if there was consent in the stories.

9. Summarize and transition to the next activity,

KEY MESSAGE:

People should always follow the rules of consent when doing sexual behaviors.

If someone breaks the rules of consent and pressures you to do something you don't want to, it is not your fault.

Next, you are going to learn what to do when someone breaks to rules of consent.

When it comes to sexual activity, people should always follow the rules of consent and only do sexual behaviors they have clear permission to do. Sometimes people break the rules and pressure or force someone to do sexual behaviors even when that person does not or cannot give consent. In the next activity we will talk about what to do if someone pressures you to do sexual behaviors you do not want to.

Remember, if someone breaks the rules of consent and pressures or forces you to do sexual touches or actions, it is NOT your fault. If this happens to you, you should tell a trusted adult to get help.

INTRODUCTION TO REFUSALS AND SCRIPTED ROLEPLAYS

PREPARING FOR THE ACTIVITY

RATIONALE

The scripted roleplay activities help students identify and practice the skills necessary to slow a situation down and provide alternative ways to clearly say No. The posters help reinforce specific refusal skills by giving students a visual reminder as they practice roleplays.

ACTIVITY LEARNING OBJECTIVE

- Recognize pressure from peers to engage in sexual activity.

MATERIALS

- Posters:
  - » *Refuse*
  - » *How to Say "NO"*
  - » *Examples of a Strong "NO"*

- Roleplays:
  - » *While They're Out* (Scripted Roleplay)
  - » *While They're Out* (Unscripted Roleplay)
- Masking tape

TIME

20–25 minutes

PROCEDURE

FACILITATOR'S NOTE

Refusal Skills and Consent:

Refusal skills are a key component of many evidence-based programs designed to reduce pregnancy, HIV and other STD among youth. Programs provide instruction and practice in delivering effective refusals, and programs including refusal skills have been shown to reduce sexual risk behaviors and increase the chances of avoiding unwanted sexual pressures.

At the same time, ideas and concepts around consent are evolving. Some institutions have adopted policies that emphasize affirmative consent, or "yes means yes," and are moving away from a "no means no" perspective. This affirmative consent approach encourages partners to communicate openly about their wishes and boundaries, both prior to and during sexual interactions. It emphasizes the risks to both parties when partners pressure each other and the responsibility of both parties to respect each other's limits.

When teaching refusal skills and evaluating the effectiveness of students' demonstration of those skills, it is important to affirm the value that no person who experiences sexual pressure, harassment or assault is to blame for being the target of those behaviors. Clear, assertive refusals can be encouraged, while also making sure youth understand that no one "deserves" to be pressured if a No is unclear.

Instruction on boundaries and respecting another person's No—both verbal and nonverbal—regardless of perceived clarity can be included to help young people understand the two-way nature of consent, and the importance of honest and respectful communication between friends and potential partners. This would be considered a "green light" adaptation and can help optimize the success of the skill building around refusals.

1. Display the *Refuse, How to Say "NO"* and *Examples of a Strong "NO"* posters.

2. Begin this activity by saying,

KEY MESSAGE:

It can be hard to talk about abstinence, but it's important that you clearly tell your partner how far you are OK with going sexually, and what you do and do not want to do.

If you're ever pressured to have sex when you don't want to, you can use something called the Refuse technique to say No.

We've talked a lot about unplanned pregnancy and STDs, but how do you say No when someone is pressuring you to have sex? Talking about abstinence can be difficult sometimes. However, it is very important that you talk with your friends or a partner about your decision to practice abstinence.

Talking openly and honestly about your decision prevents misunderstandings. We are going to work on a strategy for talking to a partner about practicing abstinence without blaming, arguing or getting into a fight. The strategy is called the Refuse technique.

3. Explain that the Refuse technique has three steps that they can use when telling a partner "No" that will make the "No" clear.

4. Review the entire *Refuse* poster with students by reading each step from the poster and describing what it means:

REFUSE

1. Say "NO." Refuse the behavior you don't want to do.

2. Explain why. Offer a reason why you don't want to do the behavior. Explaining why helps your partner understand your concerns and avoids negative reactions.

3. Suggest other activities. Provide safe alternatives to show that you still want to have a relationship with this person.

5. Explain that sometimes it can be hard to say No and stick with it, especially when it's saying No to someone you care about. Tell the class that today you are going to focus on the first step of the Refuse technique and review what it takes to say No effectively.

6. Read each characteristic on the *How to Say "NO"* poster.

HOW TO SAY "NO"

- Use and repeat the word "NO."

- Send a strong "NO" with your body language. Use hand and body gestures to make the point.

- Use a strong, serious tone of voice.

- Look directly at the person's face.

- Stand straight and tall.

- Use a serious facial expression.

7. Demonstrate how to use those characteristics by modeling the first example from the *Examples of a Strong "NO"* poster. Model by showing students how to read the example with an assertive voice and body language.

8. Next, go around the group and have each student perform an example from the chart aloud. Tell them when they say their example to say it like they mean it, and to use strong body language, tone of voice and facial expressions to make the point.

Making a Difference! For Youth with Cognitive Impairments

9. After each student says an example, ask the group to identify which characteristics the student demonstrated.

10. Compliment students on their strong refusals. Tell them the group is going to practice saying "No" some more with some roleplays.

11. Review each item of the *Refuse* poster to ensure students understand it. Tell them as they watch the roleplays they should pay attention to see if each step is used.

12. Identify a student who is a strong reader to act as Person 2 in the first roleplay; the facilitator will act as Person 1 (the pressurer). Give the student a copy of the scripted version of the *While They're Out* roleplay.

13. Begin by reading the Setting the Stage section of the roleplay. Tell the class to pay attention to whether Person 2 uses all the steps of the Refuse technique.

WHILE THEY'RE OUT – SCRIPTED ROLEPLAY

Setting the Stage: Your parents are out, and your partner comes over, hoping to have sex. You've kissed each other before, but that's as far as you want to go. You don't want to have sex. You really just want your partner to stop pressuring you.

Person 1: Why are you stopping now?

Person 2: Because I can't do this.

(continued)

(continued)

WHILE THEY'RE OUT – SCRIPTED ROLEPLAY

Person 1: It's easy. Let me help you unbutton your shirt, baby.

Person 2: No, don't. I really don't want to do this.

Person 1: Why not? Come on, I love you and I want to have sex with you.

Person 2: I know, but I don't want to have sex. This is serious.

Person 1: What are you talking about?

Person 2: I'm not ready. I don't want to have to worry about STDs or pregnancy. I have other things to think about like my goals and school. There are lots of other things we can do to show we care about each other. I hope you can understand how I feel.

Person 1: I can. It makes sense.

14. After the roleplay, thank the roleplaying student and ask them to return to their seat. Use the *Refuse* poster to process this roleplay. Point to each step on the poster and ask the group if they saw it demonstrated in the roleplay.

Try to elicit the following responses:
   » Said "No"
   » Repeated the "No"
   » Body language said "No"
   » Explained why
   » Suggested other activities

15. Ask for a new student volunteer to be Person 2 in the unscripted version of the *While They're Out* roleplay; the facilitator will again act as Person 1 (the pressurer). Tell the class that this time, Person 2 will use their own words to fill in the script. Whisper to Person 2 to be firm and to use strong body language. Again, set up the roleplay by reading the Setting the Stage section.

 Making a Difference! For Youth with Cognitive Impairments

WHILE THEY'RE OUT – UNSCRIPTED ROLEPLAY

Setting the Stage: Your parents are out, and your partner comes over, hoping to have sex. You've kissed each other before, but that's as far as you want to go. You don't want to have sex. You really just want your partner to stop pressuring you.

Person 1: Why are you stopping now?

Person 2:

Person 1: It's easy. Let me help you unbutton your shirt, baby.

Person 2:

Person 1: Why not? Come on, I love you and I want to have sex with you.

Person 2:

Person 1: What are you talking about?

Person 2:

Person 1: I can. It makes sense.

16. After the roleplay, thank the roleplaying student and ask them to return to their seat. Go over the *Refuse* poster with the class to review whether Person 2 used all the steps. Ask:

- Did Person 2 say No?

- Did the person repeat the No?

- Did the person's body language say No?

- Did the person explain why?

- Did the person suggest other activities?

17. After students respond, ask the following questions:

- Do you think this roleplay was realistic?

- What would you have done differently?

18. Compliment students' observations. Remind them that the Refuse technique will help them to say "No" when they need to. Tell them they'll have more opportunities to practice these skills in the next session.

Showing Physical Affection

Give Friendly Looks and Smiles

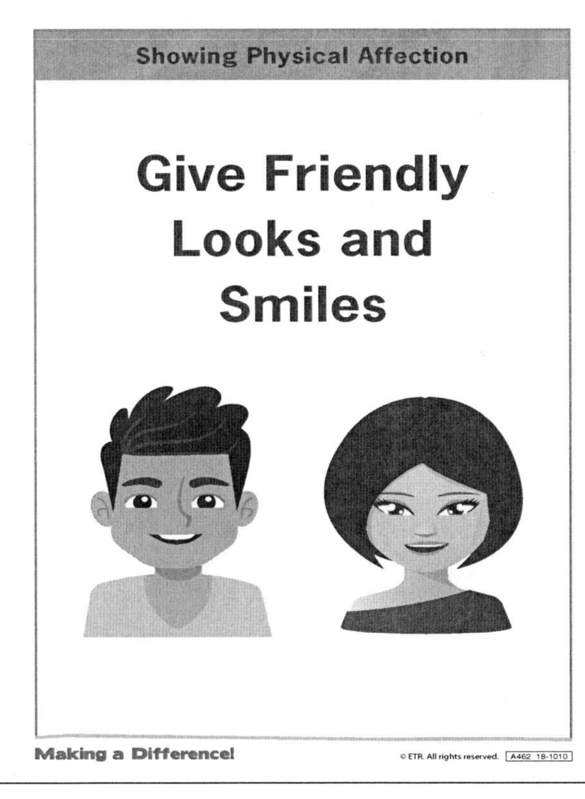

8 Posters

Consent

Consent: When both people clearly and freely agree to engage in sexual or romantic activity

Rules of consent:

- Both people must be awake, aware, and able to make decisions
- Consent can be given with words or actions
- Consent for one thing doesn't mean consent for another
- People can change their minds and take back consent at any time
- Consent must be free from pressure, tricks, bribes or threats

Poster

Refuse

1. Say "NO"

- Say "NO"
- Repeat the "NO"
- Use body language that says "NO"

2. Explain why

- Give clear reasons

3. Suggest other activities

- Offer alternatives to do

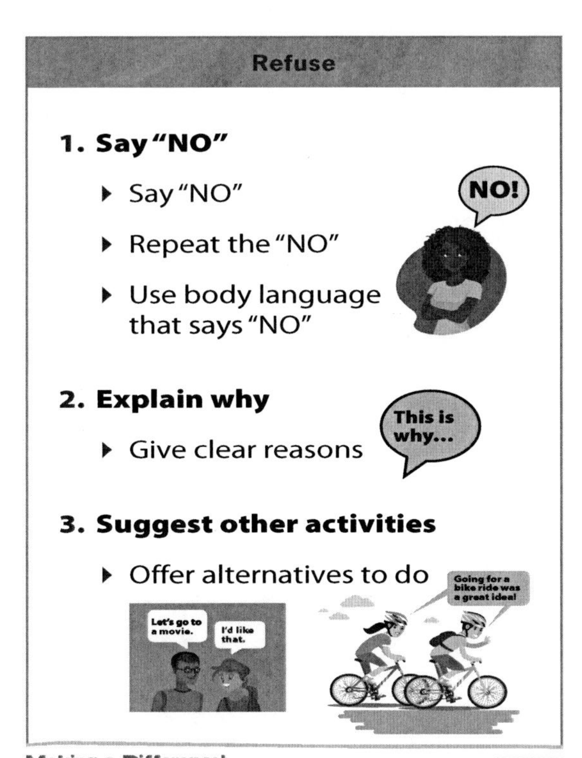

Poster

How to Say "NO"

- Use and repeat the word "NO."
- Send a strong "NO" with your body language. Use hand and body gestures to make the point.
- Use a strong, serious tone of voice.
- Look directly at the person's face.
- Stand straight and tall.
- Use a serious face.

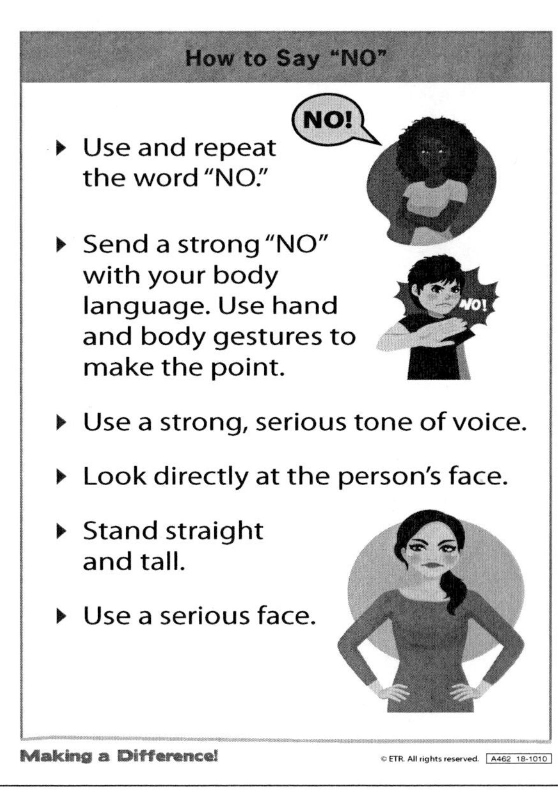

Poster

Examples of a Strong "NO"

▶ **NO!** I'm not ready to have sex yet!

▶ **NO!** I do not want to have sex!

▶ **NO!** I don't want to touch you there!

▶ **NO!** I'm not going to have sex with you!

▶ **NO!** I really mean "no"!

▶ **NO!** I do not want you to touch me there!

Making a Difference! © ETR. All rights reserved. A462 18-1010

Poster

WHILE THEY'RE OUT

Scripted Roleplay

Setting the Stage:

Your parents are out late, and your partner comes over, hoping to have sex. You've kissed each other before, but that's as far as you want to go. You don't want to have sex. You really just want your partner to stop pressuring you.

Person 1: Why are you stopping now?

Person 2: Because I can't do this.

Person 1: It's easy. Let me help you unbutton your shirt, baby.

Person 2: No, don't. I really don't want to do this.

Person 1: Why not? Come on, I love you and I want to have sex with you.

Person 2: I know, but I don't want to have sex. This is serious.

Person 1: What are you talking about?

Person 2: I'm not ready. I don't want to have to worry about STDs or pregnancy. I have other things to think about, like my goals and school. There are lots of other things we can do to show we care about each other. I hope you can understand how I feel.

Person 1: I can. It makes sense.

Making a Difference! © ETR. All rights reserved. A462 18-0911

2 Handouts

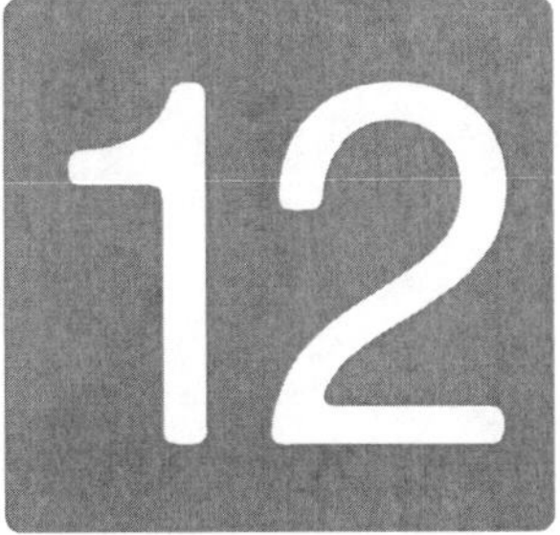

MODULE 12

ROLEPLAYS: REFUSAL AND NEGOTIATION SKILLS: PART 1

GOALS

The goals of this module are to:

- Increase students' communication, negotiation and refusal skills regarding abstinence.
- Enhance students' ability to resist situations that place them at risk for pregnancy, HIV and other STDs.
- Increase students' sense of pride and responsibility in negotiating abstinence.

LEARNING OBJECTIVES

After completing this module, students will be able to:

- Identify strategies for negotiating abstinence in romantic relationships.
- Identify and explain the characteristics of saying "NO" effectively.
- Identify and explain the body language needed for saying "NO" effectively.
- Express confidence in their ability to say "NO" in risky situations involving sexual behaviors.
- Demonstrate the ability to negotiate abstinence with a partner.

MODULE PREVIEW

The twelfth module: (1) increases students' motivation to practice abstinence; (2) builds skills to negotiate abstinence; and (3) allows students to rehearse negotiation skills and receive feedback.

STRATEGIES/METHODS

- Refuse Technique
- Roleplays

MATERIALS NEEDED — INCLUDED IN IMPLEMENTATION KIT

- Posters:
  - » *Refuse*
  - » *How to Say "NO"*
  - » *Examples of a Strong "NO"*
  - » *Explain Why*
  - » *Suggest Other Activities*
  - » *Roleplay Guidelines*

MATERIALS NEEDED — NOT INCLUDED IN IMPLEMENTATION KIT

- Masking tape

PREPARATION NEEDED

1. Hang the posters in the order they will be used.
2. Be prepared to review concepts from the eleventh module.

INSTRUCTIONAL TIME: 45–60 minutes

ACTIVITY	MINUTES NEEDED
Pre-Activity: Key Concept Review	5
A. Introduction to Refusals: Abstinence Negotiation Skills	10–15
B. Enhancing Refusals: Partner Roleplaying	30–40

 Making a Difference! For Youth with Cognitive Impairments

PREPARING FOR THE ACTIVITY

RATIONALE

Providing students with a brief review of key topics discussed in the previous module will reinforce their learning, prime them for new learning and help transition to the concepts in the upcoming module.

MATERIALS

None

TIME

5 minutes

PROCEDURE

1. Begin by writing the names of key concepts recently learned on the board:

    » Consent
    When people clearly and freely agree to engage in sexual activity. Consent must be free from pressure, tricks, bribes or threats. Another important rule for consent is that family members and helpers cannot have romantic or sexual relationships with students even if the student gives consent—it just is not allowed.

    » The Refuse Technique
    A strategy for saying No to doing a behavior or activity you don't want to do. The technique has three steps: (1) Say "NO", (2) Explain why, and (3) Suggest other activities.

2. Ask for a volunteer to explain what one of the concepts means.

3. Clarify concept if needed.

4. Check for understanding with a few other students. Repeat process with the remaining concepts.

5. Tell students that last time they practiced the first step of the Refuse technique, saying No to sexual activity they are not ready for. Tell them in this session they will learn more about the rest of the steps, and practice using the Refuse technique in some roleplays.

 Making a Difference! For Youth with Cognitive Impairments

INTRODUCTION TO REFUSALS: ABSTINENCE NEGOTIATION SKILLS

PREPARING FOR THE ACTIVITY

RATIONALE

Practicing strategies for negotiating abstinence with a partner provides students with additional skills needed to reduce their risk for unplanned pregnancy, HIV and other STDs.

ACTIVITY LEARNING OBJECTIVES

- Identify strategies for negotiating abstinence in romantic relationships.
- Identify and explain the characteristics of saying "NO" effectively.

MATERIALS

- Posters:
  - » *Refuse*
  - » *How to Say "NO"*
  - » *Examples of a Strong "NO"*
  - » *Explain Why*
  - » *Suggest Other Activities*
- Masking tape

TIME

10–15 minutes

PROCEDURE

1. Hang the *Refuse, How to Say "NO", Examples of a Strong "NO", Explain Why* and *Suggest Other Activities* posters.

2a. Introduce this activity by saying,

KEY MESSAGE:

People should always give and receive clear consent before doing sexual behaviors.

It can be hard to talk about abstinence, but it's important that you clearly tell your partner how far you are OK with going sexually to avoid confusion.

> As we learned last time, people should always follow the rules of consent and only do sexual behaviors they have clear permission to do. But sometimes people are pressured to do sexual behaviors they don't want to.
>
> Talking about abstinence can be difficult sometimes. However, it is very important that you talk with your partner about abstaining from sex. Having an open, honest discussion can help avoid misunderstandings.

2b. Tell students that the class is going to continue to practice the Refuse strategy for getting a partner to agree to not have sex, without blaming, arguing or getting into a fight.

2c. Remind them that it is never a person's fault if someone else breaks the rules of consent and pressures them to do something they don't want to do.

2d. Remind them that last time they learned about the Refuse technique and practiced the first step: Say "NO." Tell them that today they are going to review the other steps of the Refuse technique: Explain Why and Suggest Other Activities.

3. Show the *Explain Why* poster. Tell students that the Explain Why step is about giving clear reasons to support your choice. Explain that the poster shows examples of explanations they might offer for why they choose abstinence and saying No to sex.

4. Go around the group and ask each student to read aloud or repeat (for any non-readers) an example from the chart until all the examples have been spoken aloud. Instruct students to say the statements like they really mean it. Encourage students to make up their own examples as well.

EXPLAIN WHY

Give clear reasons to support your choice.

Examples:

- I want to finish school before I start having sex.

- I'm not ready for sex yet.

- I respect myself and want to protect myself by not having sex.

- Reaching my future goals is more important to me than having sex.

- I want to avoid unplanned pregnancy, HIV and other STDs.

- I have my whole life to experience sex. I'm too young right now.

- I am not ready to be a parent yet.

5. Now follow the same procedure with the *Suggest Other Activities* poster. Tell the group that the Suggest Other Activities step means to suggest another action or alternative to their partners that shows their interest in remaining close. Explain that the poster gives examples of other activities or alternative actions they might suggest instead of having sex.

6. Go around the group and ask each student to read aloud or repeat (for any non-readers) an example from the chart until all the examples have been said aloud. Instruct students to say the statements like they really mean it. Encourage students to make up their own examples as well.

PROVIDE ALTERNATIVES

Suggest another action.

Examples:

- Let's go to the movies or play a video game instead.

- Let's go to a friend's house.

- We could go get something to eat.

- I would rather do other things than have sex.

- It's a beautiful day. Let's go outside for a walk instead.

- Let's hug, talk and kiss but not have sex.

- Let's watch TV together.

- I'm thirsty. Let's get something to drink.

7. Tell students that now that they have reviewed all the steps of the Refuse technique, they are ready to practice them in roleplays in the next activity.

FACILITATOR'S NOTE

Determine the roles for the next roleplays before the activity begins. Having spent many hours with this group, you will be able to assign the roles that best facilitate learning. All students should participate.

Making a Difference! For Youth with Cognitive Impairments

ENHANCING REFUSALS: PARTNER ROLEPLAYING

PREPARING FOR THE ACTIVITY

RATIONALE

This activity offers students guided practice in negotiating abstinence with the facilitator in a controlled and safe environment. This practice increases their skills and feelings of confidence about negotiation, and the likelihood that they will use these negotiation skills in real-life situations. Those not participating directly in the roleplay have the opportunity to identify helpful strategies and coach the actors.

ACTIVITY LEARNING OBJECTIVES

- Identify strategies for negotiating abstinence in romantic relationships.
- Identify and explain the characteristics of saying "NO" effectively.
- Identify and explain the body language needed for saying "NO" effectively.
- Express confidence in their ability to say "NO" in risky situations involving sexual behaviors.
- Demonstrate the ability to negotiate abstinence with a partner.

MATERIALS

- Posters:
  - » *Roleplay Guidelines*
  - » *Refuse*
  - » *How to Say "NO"*
  - » *Examples of a Strong "NO"*
  - » *Explain Why*
  - » *Suggest Other Activities*

TIME

30–40 minutes

PROCEDURE

FACILITATOR'S NOTE

During the roleplay practice, students will be roleplaying situations with the facilitator, who may be a different or the same gender as the student. This may be awkward for straight teens who are sensitive to the suggestion of same-sex romance, for teens who identify as gay or lesbian, or

(continued)

(continued)

for teens who are transgender or gender nonconforming. It's important to address this situation directly and proactively. Here are some tips:

- Explain the situation in a matter-of-fact way. Let students know that they may be doing a roleplay with someone of a different or the same gender.

- Emphasize that they are playing roles. Doing the roleplay to practice the skill doesn't say anything about the sexual orientation of the people doing the roleplay or mean that anyone is expressing a real-life attraction toward the other person in the roleplay.

- Explain that they need to take their roles seriously because teens of all sexual orientations and gender identities need to learn how to resist sexual pressure and negotiate abstinence to protect themselves. This will help ensure that they all get the most out of the roleplay activities.

1. Post the *Roleplay Guidelines* poster before beginning this activity.

2. Introduce this activity by explaining that the class is going to practice the skills they've been learning by using them in roleplay pressure situations.

3a. Explain to students that roleplaying is a technique that can help them practice how to handle situations that are new or difficult. Tell them they should do their best to feel, sound and behave like the person they are roleplaying.

3b. Encourage them to incorporate what they have been learning about the Refuse technique. Remind them they can use the posters to help them when they are roleplaying.

4. Explain that it's important to follow some guidelines when doing roleplays. Review each item on the *Roleplay Guidelines* poster.

ROLEPLAY GUIDELINES

- Read your role carefully. Think about how that person would really behave.

- Do your best to stay in character through the whole roleplay.

- Don't let comments and laughter distract you.

(continued)

 Making a Difference! For Youth with Cognitive Impairments

(continued)

- Really try to feel and act like the person you are playing.

- Try things that you might not do ordinarily, just to see how it feels.

- Use Refuse:
  - Say NO. Repeat it. Use strong body language.
  - Explain why you don't want to engage in unsafe behavior.
  - Suggest other activities.

5. Explain to students that sometimes people don't follow the rules about consent and might pressure them to do something they don't want to do, and that they are going to practice what to do when that happens. Emphasize that the person pressuring for sexual activity in these roleplays is wrong, and that students should always follow the rules about consent.

6. If you don't have a co-facilitator, choose a student to model Roleplay A with you. The student should play the role of the person being pressured. You should play the role of the person pressuring.

7. Tell the group that they can coach the roleplayers if they get stuck. Remind them that no one says all the right things in every conversation, but we can always go back to our partners and say more about our thoughts and feelings another time.

8. Read the scenario for Roleplay A aloud, and explain the goals. Then begin the roleplay by reading the first pressure line and allowing the student to respond. Continue to pressure the student based on the scenario with 2 or 3 more pressure lines.

ROLEPLAY A

You're dating someone from another school. The two of you have decided that you're not ready to have sex. You saw your partner over the weekend and had a really good time.

It's now Monday, and your friend asks you if you had sex this weekend. You're pretty sure that your friend is having sex. At least they talk like they do. You don't know if they'll understand, but you want to tell them that you have decided to practice abstinence.

Your goal: Explain to your friend what abstinence is, and that you're choosing not to have sex.

My goal: Convince you that you should have sex.

Pressure Line: So, did you "do it" this weekend?

Allow the student to respond, and then continue the roleplay with additional pressure lines.

9. After 3–4 minutes of roleplay, review the roleplay by going over the *Refuse* poster. Encourage everyone, including the student who was roleplaying with you, to give input by asking,

- Did your classmate use the Refuse technique? How?

- Did they say No? How?

- Did they explain why? What were some of their explanations?

- Did they suggest other activities? What kinds of alternatives did they provide?

- What could they have done differently?

220

Making a Difference! For Youth with Cognitive Impairments

10. Continue to process the roleplay using one or more particularly relevant questions
     from the following list:

> - What methods/strategies did your classmate use to get the message across?
>
> - *(To student)* What pressures did your character feel?
>
> - Were there any misunderstandings or breakdowns in communication?
>
> - Did this situation seem realistic to you?
>
> - How would you have handled the situation differently?

11. Summarize Roleplay A by explaining that even when you feel good about your
     choice to practice abstinence, it doesn't mean that everyone will be supportive.
     Remind students that how they feel is most important when deciding what is right
     for them.

FACILITATOR'S NOTE

If there is time, include each student in at least one of the following roleplays. Encourage students who don't get to roleplay with you to participate in processing the roleplay and offering other ideas for refusal statements.

If you prefer and your students seem ready, you may choose to have 2 students perform together for each of the remaining roleplays, instead of having a student perform with you. Assign each student a role (i.e., person being pressured and person pressuring) and be sure to explain their goals in the roleplay.

12. Ask for a volunteer for Roleplay B. The student should play the role of the person
     being pressured. You should play the role of the person pressuring.

13. Tell the group to watch their classmate and notice whether the Refuse steps are used.
     The goal of this roleplay exercise is for the student to be proud and responsible and
     resist pressure to have sex.

Your job is to be sure that important issues in each roleplay are addressed and that students feel they can effectively use their skills. Encourage roleplaying students to be themselves, but to also pretend as if this were a real situation for them. Give suggestions and help as they need it.

You may wish to have students replay the roleplay again having the audience help out to show alternatives. What is important is that students practice communicating even when the situation is difficult. In real life, one of the hardest things to do is to fully explain yourself and be understood.

Students can also be divided into coaching groups to help each other out. This develops a cooperative atmosphere and is very energizing for the students.

14. Read the scenario for Roleplay B aloud, and then begin the roleplay by reading the first line and allowing the student to respond. Continue to pressure the student based on the scenario with 2 or 3 more pressure lines.

ROLEPLAY B

You and your partner have been hanging out for a few months. You have a lot of fun together. Sometimes you like to sit together and hold hands at the movies.

Lately, your partner has been trying to kiss and touch you when you go to the movies. You don't want to be touched that way and it makes you very uncomfortable. Your partner stops when you ask, but you think you'll have to have a serious talk about this soon.

You've just gotten back from the movies where your partner tried to kiss and touch you again. This time, your partner tells you that you have to decide whether you're going to be a couple or not.

Your goal: Convince your partner that you care for them but that you are not ready to have sex.

My goal: To convince you that dating always includes sex.

Pressure Line: Why don't you want to let me kiss you? Don't you want to be a couple?

Allow the student to respond, and then continue the roleplay with additional pressure lines.

 Making a Difference! For Youth with Cognitive Impairments

15. Review the roleplay by going over the *Refuse* poster and asking,

- Did your classmate use the Refuse technique? How?

- Did they say No? How?

- Did they explain why? What were some of their explanations?

- Did they suggest other activities? What kinds of alternatives did they provide?

- What could they have done differently?

16. Continue to process the roleplay using one or more particularly relevant questions from the following list:

- What methods/strategies did your classmate use to get the message across?

- *(To student)* What pressures was your character feeling?

- Were there any misunderstandings or breakdowns in communication?

- Were the characters able to save the relationship? If so, how? If not, why not?

- How would you have handled this situation differently?

17. Summarize Roleplay B by saying,

KEY MESSAGE:

Relationships can be challenging, especially if one person pressures the other to go further sexually than they want to go.

Talking about it can help you and your partner understand your boundaries.

If you have a partner who does not respect your boundaries, you should leave the relationship.

Relationships can be challenging at times. It gets even more complicated when one partner wants to engage in sexual intercourse and the other does not. With patience and caring, you can find a compromise that works for both of you. If you can't reach a compromise then you have to decide whether the relationship is right for you.

Remember, you are a proud and responsible person and you have goals for your future. If someone does not respect your feelings, then you need to leave the relationship, or find a partner who does.

18. Ask for a volunteer for Roleplay C. The student should play the role of the person being pressured. You should play the role of the person pressuring.

19. Tell the group to watch their classmate and notice whether the Refuse steps are used. The goal of this roleplay exercise is for the student to be proud and responsible and resist pressure to have sex.

20. Read the scenario for Roleplay C aloud, and then begin the roleplay by reading the first line and allowing the student to respond. Continue to pressure the student based on the scenario with 2 or 3 more pressure lines.

ROLEPLAY C

You invited your crush to a party, and your crush seems very excited. You're not trying to have a serious relationship right now, and you have decided to wait to have sex. You have plans for your future and an STD or pregnancy could really get in the way.

At the party, your crush starts trying to kiss and touch you. You think your crush might want to have sex, and you're feeling uncomfortable. Now, your crush is trying to convince you to be alone together upstairs.

Your goal: Convince your crush that you really care about them and explain that you do not want to have a serious relationship or sex right now.

My goal: To convince you to go upstairs and that you should have sex.

Pressure Line: Let's go upstairs. You know you want to go up there as much as I do.

Allow the student to respond, and then continue the roleplay with additional pressure lines.

21. Review the roleplay by going over the Refuse poster and asking,

- **Did your classmate use the Refuse technique? How?**

- **Did they say No? How?**

- **Did they explain why? What were some of their explanations?**

- **Did they suggest other activities? What kinds of alternatives did they provide?**

- **What could they have done differently?**

Making a Difference! For Youth with Cognitive Impairments

22. Continue to process the roleplay using one or more particularly relevant questions from the following list:

- What methods/strategies did your classmate use to get the message across?

- *(To student)* What pressures was your character feeling?

- Were there any misunderstandings or breakdowns in communication?

- Did this situation seem realistic to you?

- How would you have handled this situation differently?

23. Summarize Roleplay C by explaining that some young people decide to become sexually active for the wrong reasons—to prove themselves, to get or hold on to a partner, or because they feel insecure, lonely or curious. Tell students the healthy, proud and responsible thing to do is to look for a partner who cares about them and not just about sex.

24. Compliment students on doing a great job on the roleplays. Tell them in the next session, the class will practice some more with new roleplays.

Refuse

1. Say "NO"

- Say "NO"
- Repeat the "NO"
- Use body language that says "NO"

2. Explain why

- Give clear reasons

3. Suggest other activities

- Offer alternatives to do

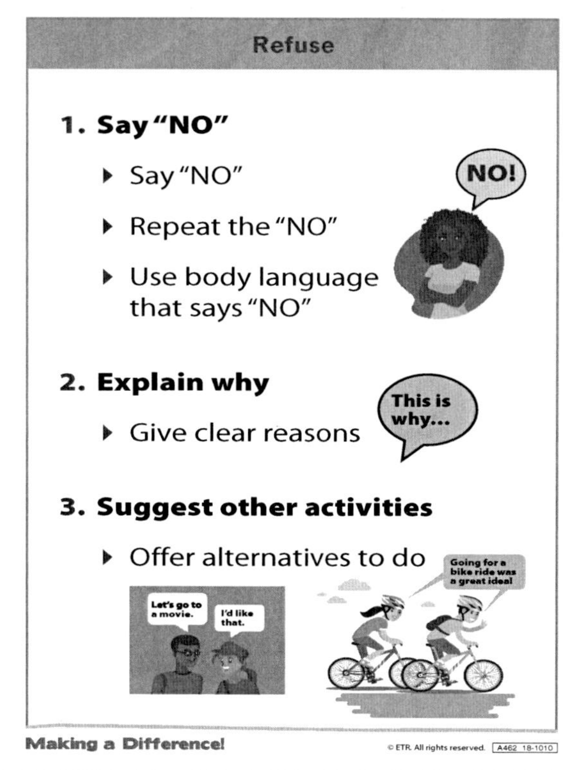

Poster

How to Say "NO"

- Use and repeat the word "NO." 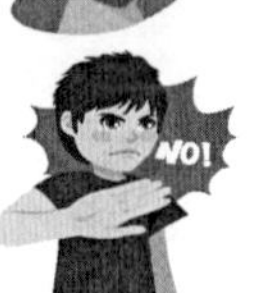

- Send a strong "NO" with your body language. Use hand and body gestures to make the point. 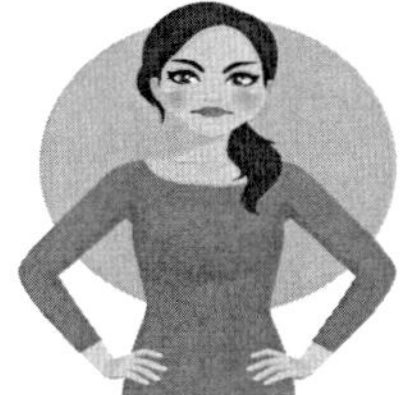

- Use a strong, serious tone of voice.
- Look directly at the person's face.
- Stand straight and tall.
- Use a serious face.

Poster

Examples of a Strong "NO"

- **NO!** I'm not ready to have sex yet!
- **NO!** I do not want to have sex!
- **NO!** I don't want to touch you there!
- **NO!** I'm not going to have sex with you!
- **NO!** I really mean "no"!
- **NO!** I do not want you to touch me there!

Poster

Explain Why

Give clear reasons to support your choice.

Examples

- I want to finish school before I start having sex.
- I'm not ready for sex yet.
- I respect myself and want to protect myself by not having sex.
- Reaching my future goals is more important to me than having sex.
- I want to avoid unplanned pregnancy, HIV and other STDs.
- I have my whole life to experience sex. I'm too young right now.
- I am not ready to be a parent yet.

Poster

   Making a Difference! For Youth with Cognitive Impairments

Suggest Other Activities

Suggest another action.

Examples

- Let's go to the movies or play a video game instead.

- Let's go to a friend's house.

- We could go get something to eat.

- I would rather do other things than have sex.

- It's a beautiful day. Let's go outside for a walk instead.

- Let's hug, talk and kiss but not have sex.

- Let's watch TV together.

- I'm thirsty. Let's get something to drink.

Poster

Roleplay Guidelines

- Listen to your role carefully. Think about how that person would really behave.

- Do your best to stay in character through the whole roleplay.

- Don't let comments and laughter distract you.

- Really try to feel and act like the person you are playing.

- Try things that you might not do ordinarily, just to see how it feels.

- Use *Refuse:*

  » **Say NO.** Repeat it. Use strong body language.

  » **Explain why** you don't want to engage in unsafe behavior.

  » Suggest **other activities.**

Poster

ROLEPLAYS: REFUSAL AND NEGOTIATION SKILLS: PART 2

GOALS

The goals of this module are to:

- Increase students' communication, negotiation and refusal skills regarding abstinence.

- Enhance students' ability to resist situations that place them at risk for pregnancy, HIV and other STDs.

- Increase students' sense of pride and responsibility in negotiating abstinence.

LEARNING OBJECTIVES

After completing this module, students will be able to:

- Identify strategies for negotiating abstinence in romantic relationships.

- Identify and explain the characteristics of saying "NO" effectively.

- Identify and explain the body language needed for saying "NO" effectively.

- Express confidence in their ability to say "NO" in risky situations involving sexual behaviors.

- Demonstrate the ability to negotiate abstinence with a partner.

- Express pride in sticking to their decision to abstain from risky sexual behaviors.

MODULE PREVIEW

The thirteenth module: (1) increases students' motivation to practice abstinence; (2) builds skills to negotiate abstinence; (3) allows students to rehearse negotiation skills and receive feedback; and (4) reinforces students' sense of pride in choosing abstinence.

STRATEGIES/METHODS

- Refuse Technique
- Roleplays
- Talking Time

MATERIALS NEEDED — INCLUDED IN IMPLEMENTATION KIT

- Posters:
  - » *Refuse*
  - » *How to Say "NO"*
  - » *Examples of a Strong "NO"*
  - » *Explain Why*
  - » *Suggest Other Activities*
  - » *Roleplay Guidelines*

MATERIALS NEEDED — NOT INCLUDED IN IMPLEMENTATION KIT

- Masking tape

PREPARATION NEEDED

1. Hang the posters in the order they will be used.
2. Be prepared to review concepts from the twelfth module.

INSTRUCTIONAL TIME: 45–60 minutes

ACTIVITY   MINUTES NEEDED

Pre-Activity: Key Concept Review   5
A. Roleplays: Refusal and Negotiation Skills 25–35
B. Talking to Your Partner About Abstinence:
   Information Review 5–10
C. Talking Time   10

PREPARING FOR THE ACTIVITY

RATIONALE

Providing students with a brief review of key topics discussed in the previous module will reinforce their learning, prime them for new learning and help transition to the concepts in the upcoming module.

MATERIALS

None

TIME

5 minutes

PROCEDURE

1. Begin by writing the names of key concepts recently learned on the board:

   » Consent
   When people clearly and freely agree to engage in sexual activity. Consent must be free from pressure, tricks, bribes or threats. Another important rule for consent is that family members and helpers cannot have romantic or sexual relationships with students even if the student gives consent—it just is not allowed.

   » The Refuse Technique
   A strategy for saying No to doing a behavior or activity you don't want to do. The technique has three steps: (1) Say "NO", (2) Explain why, and (3) Suggest other activities.

2. Ask for a volunteer to explain what one of the concepts means.

3. Clarify concept if needed.

4. Check for understanding with a few other students. Repeat process with the remaining concepts.

5.   Remind students that last time they practiced using the Refuse technique in some roleplays. Tell them that in this last session they will continue to practice the Refuse technique, and that they'll have a chance to talk about what they learned while participating in the *Making a Difference* program.

 Making a Difference! For Youth with Cognitive Impairments

PREPARING FOR THE ACTIVITY

RATIONALE

This activity allows students guided practice in negotiating abstinence with the facilitator in a controlled and safe environment. Those not participating directly in the roleplay have the opportunity to identify helpful strategies and coach those in the roleplay. This practice increases their negotiation skills, and the likelihood that they will use these negotiation skills in real-life situations.

ACTIVITY LEARNING OBJECTIVES

- Identify strategies for negotiating abstinence in romantic relationships.
- Identify and explain the characteristics of saying "NO" effectively.
- Identify and explain the body language needed for saying "NO" effectively.
- Express confidence in their ability to say "NO" in risky situations involving sexual behaviors.
- Demonstrate the ability to negotiate abstinence with a partner.

MATERIALS

- Posters:
  - » *Refuse*
  - » *Roleplay Guidelines*
- Masking tape

TIME

25–35 minutes

PROCEDURE

1. Hang the *Refuse* poster and the *Roleplay Guidelines* poster.

2. Tell students that the class is going to continue with roleplays and practicing saying No to activities that put them at risk for pregnancy and STDs.

3. Remind students that sometimes people don't follow the rules about consent, and they are practicing what to do when that happens. Emphasize that the person pressuring for sexual activity in these roleplays is wrong, and that students should always follow the rules about consent.

FACILITATOR'S NOTE

Determine the roles for the next roleplays before the activity begins. Having spent many hours with this group, you will be able to assign the roles that best facilitate learning. All students should participate.

Encourage roleplaying students to be themselves, but to also pretend as if this were a real situation for them.

For each roleplay, if you prefer and your students seem ready, you may choose to have 2 students perform together instead of having a student perform with you. Assign each student a role (i.e., person being pressured and person pressuring) and be sure to explain their goals in the roleplay.

4. Ask for a volunteer for Roleplay D. The student should play the role of the person being pressured. You should play the role of the person pressuring.

5. Tell the group to watch their classmate and notice whether the Refuse steps are used. The goal of this roleplay exercise is for the student to be proud and responsible and resist pressure to have sex.

6. Read the scenario for Roleplay D aloud, and then begin the roleplay by reading the first line and allowing the student to respond. Continue to pressure the student based on the scenario with 2 or 3 more pressure lines.

ROLEPLAY D

You and your partner have been going out for a couple of months. Your partner likes to treat you by paying for your dates and bought you some presents recently. You really enjoy all the attention and presents and your partner is a great kisser. But you don't want to go any further than kissing.

(continued)

 Making a Difference! For Youth with Cognitive Impairments

(continued)

Tonight your partner took you to a concert. When you get back to the car, your partner starts to pressure you.

Your goal: Convince your partner that you care about them and explain that you have chosen to not have sex.

My goal: To pressure you to have sex.

Pressure Line: I know you had a great time tonight and you like all the stuff I've been doing for you. Don't you think you want to do something for me in return?

Allow the student to respond, and then continue the roleplay with additional pressure lines.

7. Review the roleplay by going over the *Refuse* poster and asking,

- Did your classmate use the Refuse technique? How?

- Did they say No? How?

- Did they explain why? What were some of their explanations?

- Did they suggest other activities? What kinds of alternatives did they provide?

- What could they have done differently?

8. Continue to process the roleplay using one or more particularly relevant questions from the following list:

- What methods/strategies did your classmate use to get the message across?

- *(To student)* What pressures was your character feeling?

- Were there any misunderstandings or breakdowns in communication?

- Why shouldn't you feel pressure to give sexual favors to someone who's spent money on you or taken you out?

- How would you have handled this situation differently?

9.   Summarize Roleplay D by saying,

KEY MESSAGE:

Having sex to repay a debt or because you feel like you owe someone is not a healthy reason to have sex.

A caring partner respects your choice to wait to have sex until you are ready.

> Your sexuality is special, and you have the right to share it only with a carefully selected person once you're old enough to handle the consequences of sex. It is not a healthy choice to use sex to repay a debt. A person who cares about you will wait until you're ready and will never expect you to do something sexual that you're not ready for. Remember to be proud and responsible and make healthy sexual choices.

10.   Ask for a volunteer for Roleplay E. The student should play the role of the person being pressured. You should play the role of the person pressuring.

11.   Tell the group to watch their classmate and notice whether the Refuse steps are used. The goal of this roleplay exercise is for the student to be proud and responsible and resist pressure to have sex.

12.   Read the scenario for Roleplay E aloud, and then begin the roleplay by reading the first line and allowing the student to respond. Continue to pressure the student based on the scenario with 2 or 3 more pressure lines.

ROLEPLAY E

Your friends always seem to be talking about having sex with their partners. It makes you feel like everyone but you is having sex. They tease you about never having had sex.

You are definitely not ready to have sex yet. You want the first time to be special with someone you care a lot about.

You want to stand by the choice you made not to have sex, but you're tired of being teased by your friends. One day you walk into the gym before practice and your friend says something to tease you in front of everyone.

(continued)

Making a Difference! For Youth with Cognitive Impairments

(continued)

Your goal: Stay confident in your choice to not have sex and explain why you made that choice.

My goal: To convince you that everyone is doing it and that you should just have sex.

Pressure Line: Here comes the virgin!

Allow the student to respond, and then continue the roleplay with additional pressure lines.

13. Review the roleplay by going over the *Refuse* poster and asking,

- Did your classmate use the Refuse technique? How?

- Did they say No? How?

- Did they explain why? What were some of their explanations?

- Did they suggest other activities? What kinds of alternatives did they provide?

- What could they have done differently?

14. Continue to process the roleplay using one or more particularly relevant questions from the following list:

- What methods/strategies did your classmate use to get the message across?

- *(To student)* What pressures was your character feeling?

- How would you expect a real friend to respond if you said you had never had sex?

- Did this situation seem realistic to you?

- How would you have handled this situation differently?

15. Summarize Roleplay E by saying,

KEY MESSAGE:

Caring friends respect your healthy choices like waiting to have sex until you are ready.

Be proud and be responsible, choose your friends carefully and make the decisions that are right for you.

True friends support you when you make healthy choices for yourself. It is important to choose friends who feel similarly to you about things, or at least respect your feelings when they are different from theirs. Be proud and be responsible, choose your friends carefully and make the decisions that are right for you.

16. Ask for a volunteer for Roleplay F. The student should play the role of the person being pressured. You should play the role of the person pressuring.

17. Tell the group to watch their classmate and notice whether the Refuse steps are used. The goal of this roleplay exercise is for the student to be proud and responsible and resist pressure to have sex.

18. Read the scenario for Roleplay F aloud, and then begin the roleplay by reading the first line and allowing the student to respond. Continue to pressure the student based on the scenario with 2 or 3 more pressure lines

ROLEPLAY F

You and your partner have been dating for several months. You like each other a lot, but lately your partner has been pushing to have sex.

You do not want to have sex. You don't want to take the chance of a pregnancy or getting an STD. You get decent grades and know that could have a big impact on your plans to go to college one day. You just aren't prepared to take the risk.

The two of you are at your house one day and no one else is home. Your partner asks to go up to your bedroom. When you say that you aren't allowed to have anyone up in your room, your partner keeps pressuring you. You have to convince your partner that you really care, but you don't want to use sex to prove it.

(continued)

 Making a Difference! For Youth with Cognitive Impairments

(continued)

Your goal: Convince your partner that you care about them and explain that you are not ready and do not want to have sex.

My goal: To convince you that you should have sex.

Pressure Line: Oh, come on, your parents will never know.

Allow the student to respond, and then continue the roleplay with additional pressure lines.

19. Review the roleplay by going over the Refuse poster and asking,

- Did your classmate use the Refuse technique? How?

- Did they say No? How?

- Did they explain why? What were some of their explanations?

- Did they suggest other activities? What kinds of alternatives did they provide?

- What could they have done differently?

20. Continue to process the roleplay using one or more particularly relevant questions from the following list:

- What methods/strategies did your classmate use to get the message across?

- *(To student)* What pressures was your character feeling?

- Were there any misunderstandings or breakdowns in communication?

- Did this situation seem realistic to you?

- How would you have handled this situation differently?

21. Summarize Roleplay F by saying,

KEY MESSAGE:

Anyone can be pressured to have sex when they aren't ready to.

Sometimes people pressure their partners to have sex because they are insecure about the relationship.

Talk openly with your partner about how you feel about them and your boundaries.

Be proud and be responsible and make the decisions that are right for you.

It's not just women who are pressured to have sex. It happens to men also. It can happen to people who are straight and to people who are gay or lesbian. When people pressure other people, it's not always because they are bad or don't care about them. Sometimes they are just confused or misguided.

It takes honest and open communication to keep things balanced in a relationship. The better you can talk to your partner about your sexual thoughts and feelings, the better you can work things out. Remember, the proud and responsible thing to do is to not have sex, especially if you do not want to.

22. Ask for a volunteer for Roleplay G. The student should play the role of the person being pressured. You should play the role of the person pressuring.

23. Tell the group to watch their classmate and notice whether the Refuse steps are used. The goal of this roleplay exercise is for the student to be proud and responsible and resist pressure to have sex

24. Read the scenario for Roleplay G aloud, and then begin the roleplay by reading the first line and allowing the student to respond. Continue to pressure the student based on the scenario with 2 or 3 more pressure lines.

 Making a Difference! For Youth with Cognitive Impairments

ROLEPLAY G

You friend and crush is 2 years older and much more experienced than you. You usually do whatever they want to do, because you don't want to take the chance that they won't like you as much.

You've never had sex and you don't plan to start now. You want to wait until you finish school before you become sexually involved with someone. You know your crush feels differently about sex. That's why you avoid being alone together for more than 10 minutes at a time.

You're babysitting tonight. Right after you put the kids to sleep, the doorbell rings. It's your crush, who wants to come in for a while. You say, "I'm glad to see you but I'm not allowed visitors while I'm babysitting. You'll have to leave." But your crush keeps pressuring you.

Your goal: Tell your crush that if they really care about you, they will listen and respect you and the rules. Explain that you don't want to have sex.

My goal: To convince you to have sex.

Pressure Line: Please? It will just be for a little while.

Allow the student to respond, and then continue the roleplay with additional pressure lines.

25. Review the roleplay by going over the *Refuse* poster and asking,

- Did your classmate use the Refuse technique? How?

- Did they say No? How?

- Did they explain why? What were some of their explanations?

- Did they suggest other activities? What kinds of alternatives did they provide?

- What could they have done differently?

26. Continue to process the roleplay using one or more particularly relevant questions from the following list:

- Did the crush do anything that showed caring and respect for your classmate's character? If so, what? If not, what did the crush really care about?

- *(To student)* What pressures was your character feeling?

- Were there any misunderstandings or breakdowns in communication?

- How would you have handled the situation differently?

27. Summarize Roleplay G by saying,

KEY MESSAGE:

You never know when you might get pressured to do something.

It's important to decide how you feel about things like sex ahead of time so you can stick to your choices.

Resisting sexual pressure can be hard, but it is the proud and responsible thing to do.

You never know when you may find yourself in a pressure situation. This is why it's very important to decide in advance how you feel about things such as sex, drug use, education and your future goals. That way you can be prepared and better able to stick to your choices. Because you are a proud and responsible person, you should not let anyone, even someone you care about, pressure you to do something you've decided not to do.

28. Remind students that these roleplays showed situations where the rules of consent were not followed. Tell them that now you are going to show them what it looks like when people follow the rules of consent.

29. Ask for a volunteer to do one last roleplay. Choose one of the previous roleplay scenarios. The student should play the role of the person who is being pressured. When the student says No to the first pressure line, model respecting their choice.

30. Process the roleplay by asking,

- How was this scenario different from the others?

- *(To student)* How did it feel when your boundaries were respected?

- Where did you notice the rules of consent being followed in the roleplay? How?

Making a Difference! For Youth with Cognitive Impairments

31. Summarize the roleplay by saying,

KEY MESSAGE:

People should always follow the rules of consent when doing sexual behaviors.

Consent shows your partner you respect them.

If someone breaks the rules of consent and pressures you to do something you don't want, it is not your fault.

> When it comes to sexual activity, people should always follow the rules of consent and only do sexual behaviors they have clear permission to do. Following the rules of consent shows your partner that they are respected and avoids situations where people feel pressured or forced to do something they don't want.
>
> Remember, if someone breaks the rules of consent and pressures or forces you to do sexual touches or actions, it is NOT your fault. If this happens to you, tell a trusted adult to get help.

32a. Tell students you are impressed with how much they have learned in this program. Tell them that their roleplays show they have picked up quite a few skills, and that you hope they will remember and use these skills whenever the need arises.

32b. Then say,

KEY MESSAGE:

Healthy couples talk about the choices that are right for them.

It's important to choose partners that care about your goals, health and values.

Making proud and responsible choices, including not having sex until you are ready, will help you reach your goals for the future.

> It doesn't matter if a relationship is between a man and a woman, two women or two men. All couples have to communicate and negotiate. And all couples can make a decision to practice abstinence regardless of their sexual orientation.
>
> In a healthy relationship and when you really care about your partner, it's usually easier to talk about being abstinent. It's important to choose relationships in which both parties care about each other's goals, health and values.
>
> The proud and responsible choices that you make now can help you reach your goals for the future.

TALKING TO YOUR PARTNER ABOUT ABSTINENCE: INFORMATION REVIEW

PREPARING FOR THE ACTIVITY

RATIONALE

This activity provides tips and encouragement for applying the communication and negotiation skills that have been learned thus far, with the hope of ensuring that the knowledge, positive attitudes and skills will be translated into behavior.

ACTIVITY LEARNING OBJECTIVE

• Identify strategies for negotiating abstinence in romantic relationships.

MATERIALS

None

TIME

5–10 minutes

PROCEDURE

1. Start by saying,

KEY MESSAGE:

Abstinence from sexual activity is the surest way to avoid pregnancy and STDs.

You may have to explain to your partner why you choose to be abstinent, but a caring partner will respect your choice.

There is no doubt that abstinence is a great idea because it is the only 100 percent sure way to prevent unplanned pregnancy, HIV and other STDs. You may have to overcome a partner's reluctance to not have sex. But, if you want to abstain from sex, a caring partner will respect your decision and respect you too. You will be making a proud and responsible decision if you abstain from sex!

2. Ask students to brainstorm some suggestions that would make talking to a partner about abstinence easier. Supplement their answers with the ones below:

- Think about what you want to say ahead of time. Sort out your own feelings about abstinence before you talk with your partner.

- Choose a time to talk. The best time to discuss abstinence is before the first kiss and certainly before engaging in genital touching.

- Decide how you want to start the conversation. You might say, "I need to talk with you about something that is important to both of us," or "I've been hearing a lot lately about the consequences of sex. I feel kind of shy, but I care too much about you not to talk about this."

- Find a pamphlet or article that will help you make your point.

- Once you both agree to abstain, do something positive and fun that will help strengthen your friendship and relationship.

3. Ask students to brainstorm ways to avoid pregnancy or becoming infected with HIV or other STDs. Supplement their answers with the ones below.

- Abstain from any sexual behaviors that can cause pregnancy or transmit STDs. This includes vaginal, oral and anal sex and skin-to skin genital touching.

- Talk to your partner about HIV and other STDs.

- Educate yourself about young people and HIV.

4. Summarize what they learned from the program's activities by saying,

KEY MESSAGE:

Sex has consequences, such as pregnancy or STDs, that can get in the way of your goals. Stay focused on your goals and choose abstinence to avoid STDs and pregnancy.

We have covered a lot of information in this program. It is important to remember that getting pregnant or getting someone pregnant before you are able to care for a child, or getting HIV or other STDs, can have far-reaching consequences for you, your partner, your friends, your family and your community.

You can be proud and responsible by making healthy decisions, including abstaining from sex. You can also encourage other young people to do the same.

Remember: abstinence is the only 100 percent sure way of preventing unplanned pregnancy, HIV and other STDs.

FACILITATOR'S NOTE

If you have time following this activity, you may want to consider leading the "Healthy Relationships" activity in Appendix A to reinforce the characteristics of healthy relationships.

Making a Difference! For Youth with Cognitive Impairments

TALKING TIME

PREPARING FOR THE ACTIVITY

RATIONALE

This activity provides students a sense of closure to the program.

ACTIVITY LEARNING OBJECTIVE

• Express pride in sticking to their decision to abstain from risky sexual behaviors.

MATERIALS

None

TIME

10 minutes

PROCEDURE

1. Ask each student to share something learned in the group that will help in achieving goals for the future.

2. Thank students for their attendance and let them know how much you enjoyed working with them.

3. Summarize the activity by saying,

KEY MESSAGE:

Remember that abstinence, or not having sex, is the only 100 percent sure way to avoid pregnancy and STDs.

Stay focused on your goals, and make the proud and responsible decisions that are right for you.

Those were good responses. I am very proud of each and every one of you. Thank you for being part of this program. Now you can teach your friends and family what you've learned here.

We have spent a lot of time together talking about making proud and responsible sexual decisions and the surest way to protect yourselves. Remember everything you learned, and don't forget that practicing abstinence is the only 100 percent sure way to keep yourself safe from unplanned pregnancy, HIV and other STDs.

Making a Difference! For Youth with Cognitive Impairments

Refuse

1. Say "NO"

- Say "NO"
- Repeat the "NO"
- Use body language that says "NO"

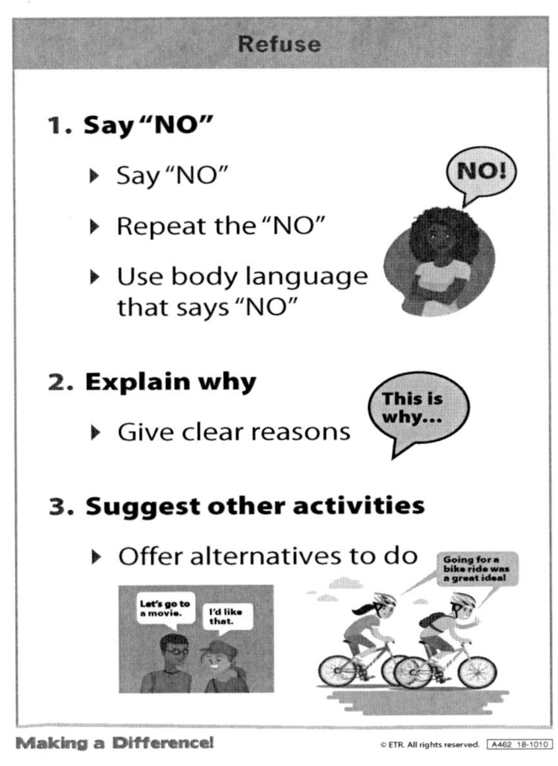

2. Explain why

- Give clear reasons

3. Suggest other activities

- Offer alternatives to do

Poster

How to Say "NO"

- Use and repeat the word "NO." 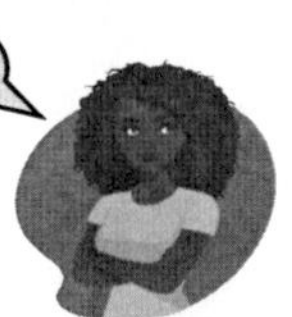

- Send a strong "NO" with your body language. Use hand and body gestures to make the point. 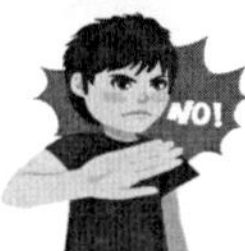

- Use a strong, serious tone of voice.

- Look directly at the person's face.

- Stand straight and tall. 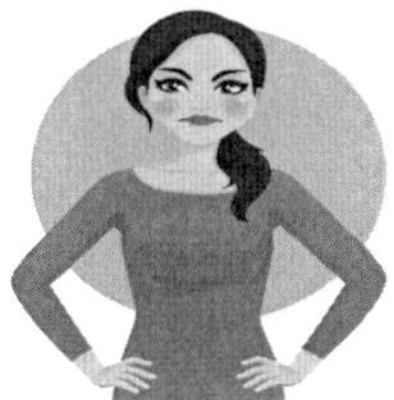

- Use a serious face.

Poster

Examples of a Strong "NO"

- **NO!** I'm not ready to have sex yet!
- **NO!** I do not want to have sex!
- **NO!** I don't want to touch you there!
- **NO!** I'm not going to have sex with you!
- **NO!** I really mean "no"!
- **NO!** I do not want you to touch me there!

Poster

Explain Why

Give clear reasons to support your choice.

Examples

- I want to finish school before I start having sex.
- I'm not ready for sex yet.
- I respect myself and want to protect myself by not having sex.
- Reaching my future goals is more important to me than having sex.
- I want to avoid unplanned pregnancy, HIV and other STDs.
- I have my whole life to experience sex. I'm too young right now.
- I am not ready to be a parent yet.

Poster

Suggest Other Activities

Suggest another action.

Examples

- Let's go to the movies or play a video game instead.
- Let's go to a friend's house.
- We could go get something to eat.
- I would rather do other things than have sex.
- It's a beautiful day. Let's go outside for a walk instead.
- Let's hug, talk and kiss but not have sex.
- Let's watch TV together.
- I'm thirsty. Let's get something to drink.

Making a Difference!

 A462 18-1010

Poster

Roleplay Guidelines

- Listen to your role carefully. Think about how that person would really behave.
- Do your best to stay in character through the whole roleplay.
- Don't let comments and laughter distract you.
- Really try to feel and act like the person you are playing.
- Try things that you might not do ordinarily, just to see how it feels.
- Use *Refuse:*
  - » **Say NO.** Repeat it. Use strong body language.
  - » **Explain why** you don't want to engage in unsafe behavior.
  - » Suggest **other activities.**

Making a Difference!

 A462 18-1010

Poster

Making a Difference! For Youth with Cognitive Impairments

Making a Difference!

For Youth with Cognitive Impairments

FIFTH EDITION

APPENDIXES

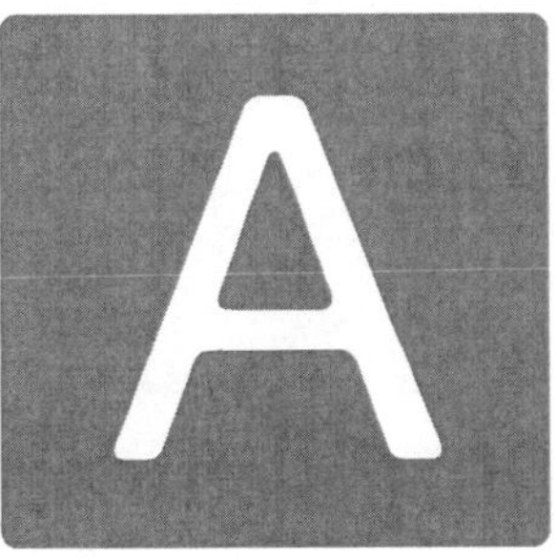

ADDITIONAL GAMES/ACTIVITIES

The information in the sections that follow should be viewed as supplemental. The authors encourage use of this section when you are attempting to address issues and needs that may emerge in the group.

Appendix A provides additional roleplays that integrate varying sexual orientations. Two games, AIDS Basketball and HIV/STD Jeopardy, have also been provided as a fun way to review HIV information. There are also several activities provided to cover basic information about puberty, private and public spaces, and healthy relationships.

Table of Contents

ADDITIONAL ROLEPLAY SITUATIONS/ABSTINENCE

FACILITATOR'S NOTE

The following roleplays are additional situations that you might wish to use during the roleplays.

ROLEPLAY 1: TARYN AND TANYA

Theme: Two females; STD/HIV concerns in a lesbian relationship; abstinence

Observe: TARYN using the Refuse technique

Taryn

You have just started your first sexual relationship with Tanya. You are not sure if two women involved in a sexual relationship have to worry about STDs, including HIV. You do not want to have sex. You would rather hold hands, kiss and body rub.

Your role: Tell Tanya that you don't want to have sex.

Tanya

You and Taryn have been dating for two weeks. You like Taryn a lot. You have never thought about STDs or HIV. You hope Taryn wants to take this relationship to another level and have sex with you.

Summarize Roleplay 1 by saying,

KEY MESSAGE:

It is important to talk with your partner about your sexual boundaries.

Abstinence is the surest way to avoid STDs.

Communication is the most important aspect of any relationship no matter what your sexual orientation. The more knowledge and understanding you have, the better able you are to protect yourself. Remember that abstinence is the only 100 percent effective way to protect yourself from STDs, including HIV.

ROLEPLAY 2: ALONZO AND WILL

Theme: Two males; HIV and abstinence

Observe: ALONZO using the Refuse technique

Alonzo

You really like Will. You feel you are too young to have sex. You have goals and dreams for the future. You want to wait.

Your role: Get Will to agree that it is better to wait to have sex.

Will

You and Alonzo have just started dating. You have never used condoms to protect yourself during sex because you think you are too young to get HIV. You think only older guys get HIV and that young ones are safe. You really like Alonzo and want to have sex with him.

Summarize Roleplay 2 by saying,

KEY MESSAGE:

Anyone can get HIV.

Abstinence is the surest way to protect yourself from STDs like HIV.

People are at risk for HIV infection regardless of whether they are straight, gay or bisexual, young or old. It's better if you know who you are and what you want out of life before you get involved with anyone sexually. Remember, abstaining from sex is the surest way to protect yourself from STDs, including HIV.

ROLEPLAY 3: DIANE AND LAUREN

Theme: Concerns about HIV and STDs when one partner is bisexual; abstinence

Observe: LAUREN using the Refuse technique

Lauren

You really, really like Diane. She is your second girlfriend. You know Diane has had unprotected sex with men before. You just aren't ready to have sex with her yet. You have concerns about HIV and other STDs.

Your role: Talk to Diane about your concerns, tell her that you are not ready to have sex.

Diane

You have had sex with guys; sometimes you had unprotected sex (no condoms). Lauren is your first female partner. You care for Lauren a lot. You feel no one understands you like she does. Lauren excites you and you want to have sex with her.

Summarize Roleplay 3 by saying,

KEY MESSAGE:

Abstinence is the surest way to protect yourself from STDs like HIV.

It is important to communicate with your partner about your sexual boundaries.

Everyone who has unprotected sex is at risk for HIV infection. Abstaining from sex is the only way to be 100 percent sure you will not contract HIV or other STDs. Discuss your decision to abstain from sex with your partner. Communication is the key to a good relationship.

Making a Difference! For Youth with Cognitive Impairments

ROLEPLAY 4: COURT AND ASH

Theme: One partner wants to abstain; they discuss their options

Observe: COURT using the Refuse technique

Court

You and Ash have been dating for many months and have talked about having sex. You have kissed, hugged and grinded (rubbed your bodies together). You are not ready to have sex yet. Ash is becoming impatient and wants to have sex with you.

Your role: Tell Ash that you want to abstain from having sex, and explain why.

Ash

You have been dating Court for many months. You are in love and want to have sex to show how you feel. You are tired of kissing, hugging and grinding, getting excited and then nothing. Court wants to talk to you after school. You are ready to have sex and you are going to tell Court what you want.

Summarize Roleplay 4 by saying,

KEY MESSAGE:

It is important to communicate with your partner about your sexual boundaries.

Abstinence is the surest way to avoid STDs.

It is important to talk about your decision to abstain from sex before you are in the heat of the moment. Be confident in your decision. Discuss other ways of being intimate such as holding hands, kissing, hugging, etc. Remember, the only way to be 100 percent sure that you will not get HIV or another STD through sexual contact is to abstain from sex.

THE AIDS BASKETBALL GAME*

PREPARING FOR THE ACTIVITY

RATIONALE

This activity is a way to review and reinforce the information about HIV transmission covered in this program. It also allows you to end the class with a fun and high-energy activity.

MATERIALS

- Markers
- Newsprint
- Masking tape
- AIDS Basketball Questions (included in activity)

TIME

20–30 minutes

PROCEDURE

1. Tell the group you're going to play "AIDS basketball," a game to review what everybody has learned about HIV and AIDS.

2. Divide the group into two teams.

3. Start by giving the rules,

> - Each team will get the chance to answer a question.
>
> - Take turns so that each team member gets a chance to answer a question.
>
> - The other team members can help, but the answer must be given within 20 seconds.

(continued)

* "AIDS Basketball" from *AIDS: What Young Adults Should Know*, 2nd ed., by William L. Yarber. Adapted with permission from the Association for the Advancement of Health Education.

- Only correct answers earn points. Correct answers are worth two or three points.

- The team members answering the question can choose whether they want a two- or three-point question.

- If the answer is wrong or not given in time, I will give the correct answer and the other team will get a foul shot (a one-point question).

4. Keep score on the board or on newsprint.

5. Try to get through all the questions but remember you have only 20-30 minutes. The game goes quickly and is stimulating.

FACILITATOR'S NOTE

If no one is given a foul shot, use the foul questions in the game for one point each.

6. Use the questions that follow for the game. Correct answers are provided. Correct answers for True and False questions are in parentheses.

7. At the end of the game total the team scores and declare a winning team.

8. Acknowledge students for remembering a lot of information about HIV. Encourage them to use the strategies they have learned to make proud and responsible decisions.

AIDS BASKETBALL
QUESTIONS AND ANSWERS

TWO-POINT QUESTIONS

1. **What does AIDS stand for?**

    - Acquired immunodeficiency syndrome

2. **What causes AIDS?**

    - HIV, the human immunodeficiency virus

3. **Which body system does HIV damage?**

    - Immune system

4. **What happens to a person with AIDS that usually does not happen to people with a healthy immune system?**

    - They get certain rare diseases called opportunistic infections.

5. **Name three of the body fluids through which HIV is transmitted.**

    - Semen, vaginal secretions, rectal (bottom) fluids, blood and breast milk (any 3)

6. **What are the most common ways HIV is transmitted?**

    - Unprotected sexual intercourse and exchange of blood

7. **What drug-related behavior allows the exchange of blood?**

    - Sharing needles

8. **How do most children get infected with HIV?**

    - From their infected mothers during pregnancy, at birth or through breastfeeding

9. **(True) or False. Anyone who has unprotected sex or shares needles can get HIV.**

10. **(True) or False. Anal sex increases your chances of getting HIV.**

11. **True or (False). There is now a cure for AIDS.**

12. **(True) or False. Performing oral sex increases the chance of getting HIV.**

 Making a Difference! For Youth with Cognitive Impairments

13. True or (False). You can catch HIV like you catch a cold, because HIV can be carried in the air.

14. (True) or False. Sexual abstinence is the only 100 percent sure way to prevent pregnancy and sexually transmitted diseases.

THREE-POINT QUESTIONS

15. **What are two ways to prevent HIV?**
    - Abstinence
    - Not sharing needles

16. **Name three ways HIV is passed.**
    - During unprotected sex
    - By sharing needles and syringes
    - From an infected woman to her fetus or newborn child

17. **Name three types of sex that can pass HIV.**
    - Anal sex
    - Vaginal sex
    - Oral sex

18. **(True) or False. People without any symptoms can have HIV and pass it to a sexual partner.**

19. **True or (False). The only reason people practice abstinence is because of religious beliefs.**

20. **Name three sexual behaviors that do not involve body fluids that can carry HIV. (Any 3)**
    - Hugging
    - Massage
    - Touching
    - Masturbation
    - Sexual fantasy
    - Grinding
    - Romantic talking
    - Cuddling

21. **Name two things that can make practicing abstinence easier. (Any 3)**
    - knowing why you want to practice abstinence
    - telling your friends about your choice to abstain
    - talking to your partner about your choice early in the relationship
    - avoiding risky situations
    - knowing your physical limits

FOUL SHOOTING QUESTIONS (ONE POINT)

22. **Yes or No. Which of these can transmit HIV?**

Stress	no
Dry kissing	no
Sharing needles with someone who is HIV positive	yes
Touching someone who has HIV	no
Using the same fork as someone who is HIV positive	no
Using someone's comb	no
Being around someone with AIDS	no

23. **(True) or False. People can have HIV and give it to others even if they do not look or feel sick.**

24. **True or (False). You cannot get HIV from sex if you have sex with only one person during your whole life.**

25. **True or (False). People infected with HIV through injecting drugs are not likely to pass the virus to sex partners unless the partner also injects drugs.**

Making a Difference! For Youth with Cognitive Impairments

HIV/STD JEOPARDY

PREPARING FOR THE ACTIVITY

RATIONALE

Using a familiar game format that is popular and fun will enhance student learning of HIV-related facts and/or serve as a review of the facts.

MATERIALS

- HIV/STD Jeopardy Questions
- Board for keeping score

TIME

15–30 minutes

PROCEDURE

1. Explain that the activity will reinforce information covered so far. It is a game called *HIV/STD Jeopardy*.

FACILITATOR'S NOTE

Explain that in the real game of Jeopardy, the contestants receive an answer and must come up with the correct question. In HIV/STD Jeopardy, students will be asked a question and then must come up with the correct answer.

2. Divide the group into two teams.

3. One person from each team chooses a category and a point value. If he or she gets the correct answer, the team receives the points. If not, the other team has the opportunity to confer, reply and earn the points.

4. The next team has the chance to choose a category and a point value. The game continues until the board is cleared and the game is over. The team with the highest number of points wins the game.

5. Have someone keep score on a sheet of paper or on the board.

6. At the end of the game, acknowledge students for remembering a lot of information about HIV. Remind them that they have learned many strategies in this program that they can use to help keep themselves safer.

Making a Difference! For Youth with Cognitive Impairments

HIV/STD JEOPARDY QUESTIONS

HIV FACTS

$100

What does AIDS stand for?

- Acquired immunodeficiency syndrome

$200

What is HIV?

- The virus that causes AIDS

$300

Who can get HIV?

- Anyone. It's not who you are but what you do. People are not high risk, but their actions may be.

$400

What system does HIV affect?

- The immune system

$500

What happens to a person with HIV that usually does not occur in people with a healthy immune system?

- They acquire certain rare diseases.

STD FACTS

$100

What does STD stand for?

- Sexually transmitted disease

$200

Name 3 STDs.

- Syphilis, HPV, herpes, gonorrhea, trichomoniasis, chlamydia, HIV, hepatitis B

$300

Name 2 symptoms of STDs.
- Burning when urinating (or peeing), unusual fluids from the penis/vagina, sores, bumps, itching, rash. Sometimes there are no symptoms.

$400

What is the difference between a curable STD and a treatable STD?

- People can take medicine to make a curable STD go away. Treatable STDs can be treated, but the STD stays in the body.

$500

What happens if a person does not get treated for an STD?

- It can lead to other health problems, such as pelvic inflammatory disease, sterility, blindness, death.

Making a Difference! For Youth with Cognitive Impairments

PREVENTION

$100

What are two ways to prevent the spread of HIV?

- Abstinence and not sharing needles

$200

True or False: The only reason people practice abstinence is because of religious beliefs.

- False

$300

Name two high-risk behaviors.

- Unprotected anal, oral or vaginal sex, sharing needles

$400

What are the steps in the Refuse Technique for preventing an unsafe situation?

- Say NO, Explain Why, Provide Alternatives, Talk It Out

$500

What are some safe sexual behaviors that won't spread HIV or other STDs?

- Kissing, massage (with clothes on), masturbation, fantasy

TRANSMISSION

$100

Name two ways that HIV is spread.

- Unprotected sex, sharing needles, from mother to fetus during pregnancy or childbirth, from mother to child through breastfeeding

$200

What are two ways you cannot get HIV?

- Sharing drinking glasses, touching, sitting in a classroom together, toilet seats, other casual contact

$300

Name two body fluids that can spread HIV.

- Blood, semen, vaginal secretions, rectal (bottom) fluids, breast milk

$400

How were most children with HIV infected?

- From mother to fetus during pregnancy, at birth, or through breast milk

$500

Why is early treatment for HIV important?

- There is no cure for HIV, but anti-retroviral treatments (ART) can be started while the person still feels healthy. If people with HIV remain in medical care and continue to take the medicines to keep low viral loads, they can live long, healthy lives.

Making a Difference! For Youth with Cognitive Impairments

ABSTINENCE FACTS

$100

What is the surest way to prevent the spread of HIV/ STD?

- Abstinence

$200

True or False. People practicing abstinence can still have oral sex.

- False. Abstinence means not having anal, vaginal or oral sex. It also means not engaging in skin-to-skin genital touching that could spread certain STDs (herpes, syphilis, HPV).

$300

Name two things that can make practicing abstinence easier.

- Knowing why you want to practice abstinence (or not have sex), telling your friends about your choice to abstain, talking to your partner about your choice early in the relationship, avoiding risky situations, knowing your physical limits

$400

What is the difference between practicing abstinence and never having had sex?

- Practicing abstinence means choosing not to have sex. A person who has had sex in the past can decide to stop having sex and be abstinent. Anyone who chooses not to engage in any sexual activities that could cause pregnancy or transmit HIV or other STD is practicing abstinence.

$500

Name two benefits of abstaining from sex.

- Can help you reach your goals; protects you from unplanned pregnancy; allows you to avoid STDs, including HIV; can feel proud of yourself for making a responsible choice; can make your family proud; can get to know a partner well and do other fun things

PUBERTY AND ADOLESCENT SEXUAL DEVELOPMENT DISCUSSION

PREPARING FOR THE ACTIVITY

RATIONALE

Having the participants review the physical and emotional aspects of puberty and sexual development will give them a better understanding of their growth and development.

MATERIALS

- Body Changes poster
- Optional posters:
  - » *Female Body—Inside*
  - » *Female Body—Outside*
  - » *Male Body—Inside*

TIME

20–30 minutes

PROCEDURE

1. Tell the group that you are going to discuss puberty, sexual development, and tips on proper hygiene.

2. Explain to students that puberty is when a person first becomes capable of sexual reproduction—or making babies—and many changes begin to take place within the body and a person's emotions.

3. Display the *Body Changes* poster.

FACILITATOR'S NOTE

You may choose to display the optional *Female Body* and *Male Body* posters. These 3 posters can be used for reference during your discussion or while answering student questions, or they may be used to review the basic anatomical structures of the genitals and reproductive systems.

4. Review the contents of the *Body Changes* poster by asking the following questions. Remind students that they can use the poster to answer the questions.

>   What are the body changes of puberty for girls?

    -   **Answers:** breasts develop; underarm hair; hips develop; body fills out; menstruation; acne; sweat more actively; voice changes; pubic hair, other body hair; muscles develop

>   What are the body changes of puberty for boys?

    -   **Answers:** breasts swell (a little); underarm hair, facial hair; testicles, scrotum, penis develop; sperm are made; acne; sweat more actively; voice changes; pubic hair, other body hair; muscles develop

>   How old do you think girls are usually when puberty begins?

    -   **Answer:** As early as 9 or as late as 16

>   How old do you think boys are usually when puberty begins?

    -   **Answer:** As early as 9 or as late as 16

FACILITATOR'S NOTE

It is very important to discuss the wide variation of ages when puberty can begin and progress. Girls generally begin puberty earlier than boys.

Puberty can begin as early as age 9 or as late as age 16 and still be completely normal.

5. Next, remind students that there are emotional changes that young people feel as they become teenagers. Ask them what they think are some of the emotional changes that teens go through.

    Answers:

    >   Need for independence (for example, making their own decisions and doing things on their own), desire to be accepted by peers, rebellion against authority, mood swings, feeling nervous about changes, excitement about changes, hopes and dreams for the future

    If students have trouble answering the question, provide them some examples.

6. Tell the group that another part of puberty is proper hygiene.

7. Ask the following questions. Use the information under the questions to provide
    information during your discussion.

» Can you think of some hygiene needs for girls during puberty?

Answers include:

– Wipe from front to back after using the bathroom.

– Wear cotton underwear.

– Change tampons/pads frequently when menstruating.

– Do not douche or use feminine hygiene products because they can cause irritation.
   Vaginas are self-cleaning; they are not dirty.

– Wash daily and use underarm deodorant.

– Wash face gently with mild soap.

– Don't touch your face often.

– Don't pop or squeeze pimples.

– If your skin is oily, use an astringent to dry it out, but don't overuse it. Your skin may
   react by producing even more oil.

– Drink lots of water, eat well, and get lots of rest.

» Can you think of some hygiene needs for boys during puberty?

Answers include:

– Wash carefully under foreskin (if applicable).

– Wash daily and use underarm deodorant.

– Wash face gently with mild soap.

– Don't touch your face often.

– Don't pop or squeeze pimples.

– If your skin is oily, use an astringent to dry it out, but don't overuse it. Your skin may
   react by producing even more oil!

– Drink lots of water, eat well, and get lots of rest.

» Do we see anything in common for boys and girls regarding hygiene?

Answers:

– Wash daily and use underarm deodorant.

– Wash face gently with mild soap.

– Don't touch your face often.

Making a Difference! For Youth with Cognitive Impairments

– Don't pop or squeeze pimples.

– If your skin is oily, use an astringent to dry it out, but don't overuse it. Your skin may react by producing even more oil!

– Drink lots of water, eat well, and get lots of rest.

» Why do many teens have perspiration odors and get pimples?

Answer:

– They have more sweat production, more oil production, and are having hormone changes. All these things make it easier for everyday germs to grow. Body odor is caused when everyday germs grow in warm, moist areas. So teens should wash daily and use deodorant.

» Do adolescents care about their appearance? (YES) Why?

» Do they care about their hair, body odor, breath and clothes?

» Do you care about these things for yourself?

» What do you do about them?

» What does this have to do with your health?

8. **Summarize by saying,**

KEY MESSAGE:

Puberty, the changes to the body and emotions that happens as young people become teenagers, happens between age 9 and 16.

Taking care of your body and using proper hygiene is the proud and responsible thing to do.

> **It is very important to know the wide range of ages when puberty can begin and progress. Girls generally begin puberty earlier than boys. Puberty can begin as early as age 9 or as late as age 16 and still be completely normal. The proud and responsible thing to do is know your body and take care of it. Respect and protect it. You won't get another one.**

THE PUBERTY KIT*

PREPARING FOR THE ACTIVITY

RATIONALE

This activity is a fun way to introduce youth to various hygiene and personal care products that can help them deal with bodily functions and changes related to puberty.

MATERIALS

- Bag or box large enough to hold several items
- Various puberty-related hygiene and personal care products, such as:
  » **Hair care:** comb, brush, shampoo
  » **Dental care:** toothbrush, toothpaste, dental floss, mouthwash
  » **Odor control:** various types of deodorant/antiperspirant
  » **Body cleansing:** soap, body wash, hand sanitizer, wipes
  » **Feminine hygiene:** maxi-pad, mini-pad, tampon
  » **Body hair:** razor, shaving cream
  » **Miscellaneous:** nail clippers, laundry detergent

TIME

20–30 minutes

PROCEDURE

1. Begin this activity by explaining to the group that it's important to practice proper hygiene and to take care of your body, especially when going through the changes of puberty.

2. Tell the group that the class is going to explore a "Puberty Kit," which is a fun way to look at and talk about personal care and hygiene products that can help them address changes to their body related to puberty.

* Adapted with permission from materials provided by Kent Intermediate School District.

3. **Explain the game rules:**

   » You will walk around the room with the Puberty Kit, allowing each student to reach in and take an item. Participation is voluntary, and a student may decline to take an item.

   » After a student takes an item, the student will explain to the class what the item is, how it is used, and why it might be in the bag. If the student who took the item does not know the answers, you will ask for volunteers to help answer the questions.

   » You will then lead a brief class discussion of the item and why it might be useful or necessary. For example, puberty can cause you to sweat more and have body odor, so it is important to keep your body and clothes clean and smelling fresh.

FACILITATOR'S NOTE

When needed, be sure to reframe students' explanations so messages about items are general and not shaming or imposing gender stereotypes.

For example, if a student were to say that razors are for girls to shave their underarms to avoid odor, the facilitator should reframe by explaining that while hair under the arms can contribute to odor for anyone, it can be managed by cleaning under the arms and using deodorant daily, and that girls can shave their underarms if and when they decide they want to.

4. **Try to get through all of the items in the kit. The game goes quickly and is a good way to stimulate discussion.**

5. **At the end of the game, praise the group for what they knew and learned about how to practice good hygiene and keep their bodies and clothing clean and smelling fresh.**

PREPARING FOR THE ACTIVITY

RATIONALE

This activity is a fun way to help youth understand the difference between public and private spaces and where it may be appropriate or inappropriate to engage in certain behaviors.

MATERIALS

- *Public or Private Places* poster
- *Public or Private Bingo* card for each student
- A baggie for each student containing items to use as markers on the Bingo card (e.g., coins, beans or other small items)

TIME

20–30 minutes

PROCEDURE

1. Display the *Public or Private Places* poster. Introduce this activity by explaining to the group that they are going to learn the difference between public and private.

2. Ask students if they know what a public place is, and solicit answers from volunteers.

3. Explain that public places are those where other people are with you or could join you. Give examples such as a classroom, school bus, park, store, public restroom, or a room in a house without a closed door to keep others out. Point out the examples on the poster.

4. Next, ask the group if they know what a private space is, and solicit answers from volunteers.

* Adapted with permission from materials provided by Kent Intermediate School District.

5. Explain that private places are those where other people are prevented from entering. Give examples such as their bedroom or bathroom at home with the door closed and locked. Point out the examples on the poster.

6. Explain that in addition to public and private places, there are public and private behaviors.

7. Remind the group public places are those where other people could enter any time. Explain that this means it's important to only do behaviors that are OK to do around other people in these places. Tell them these are things like eating, talking and reading a book.

8. Tell the group that private behaviors, such as brushing your teeth, getting dressed or undressed, bathing, and touching your genitals (masturbating), are things that should only be done in private places.

9. Reemphasize that in public places, it's very important never to touch their genitals or another person's genitals, remove their clothing or another person's clothing, or masturbate because it could make other people upset or embarrassed. Tell them it is OK to engage in some romantic behaviors in public places such as kissing, hugging and holding hands, but only if the other person agrees to these activities.

10. Tell the group that now you are going to play "Public/Private Bingo" to practice telling the difference between public and private places.

11. Explain the game rules:

    - Each person will get a Bingo card and a baggie with items to mark the card.

    - The Bingo cards have pictures of different types of places, such as a public restroom, a bedroom and a classroom.

    - Explain that you will call out the name of a place, and then ask students if it is a public or private place. Tell them they can use the poster to help decide if a place is public or private.

    - If a student has a picture of that place on the Bingo card, then they place a marker on the picture.

    - This process will continue until someone has a Bingo (4 marked pictures in a horizontal, vertical or diagonal line). When someone has Bingo, they should say "Bingo!"

    - The game will then start again. The person who had Bingo clears their card, but the rest of the group keep the markers on their card.

12. Distribute the Bingo cards and marker items.

13. When you call out each place, describe it or tell a little story about it to help the group determine if it is a public or private place.

14. As students answer if it is a public or private place, reinforce the correct response and what types of behaviors are OK and not OK to be done there.

15. When you are ready to stop the game, praise the group for learning a lot about public and private places and what activities are OK to do there. Ask the group if they have any questions about public or private places or behaviors.

BINGO CARD LOCATIONS

Note: be sure to mix up the order of the locations you describe as the game continues.

- Bathroom at home (with tub)
- Bathroom at home (with shower)
- Beach
- Bed
- Bedroom
- Classroom
- Grocery store
- Living room
- Mall
- Park
- Pet store
- Playground
- Public restroom
- Restaurant
- School bus
- Swimming pool

Making a Difference! For Youth with Cognitive Impairments

HEALTHY RELATIONSHIPS

PREPARING FOR THE ACTIVITY

RATIONALE

By identifying characteristics of healthy and unhealthy relationships, students will be able to distinguish the differences. Many teens aren't clear about behaviors that are unhealthy in relationships, believing for example, that extreme jealousy is normal and a sign of love.

MATERIALS

- Markers
- *TREO: Four Parts of a Healthy Relationship* poster
- Pre-labeled newsprint:
  - » *Signs of Healthy Relationships*
  - » *Signs of Unhealthy Relationships*

TIME

20–30 minutes

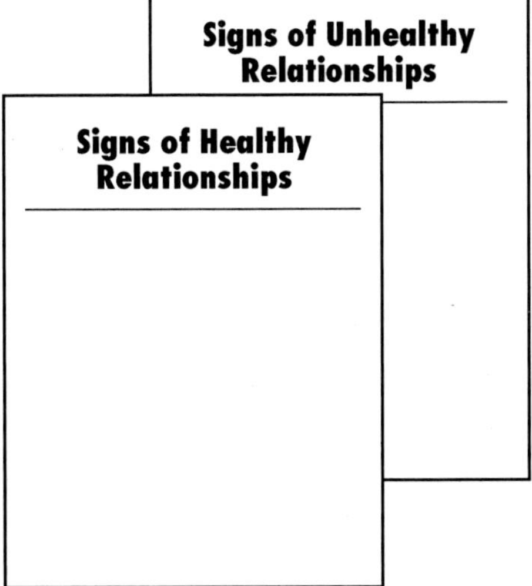

PROCEDURE

1. Introduce the activity by asking the group to think about what is needed for a healthy relationship.

2. Ask the group what they think the signs or qualities of a healthy relationship are. Solicit responses from the group and record their answers on the pre-labeled newsprint.

FACILITATOR'S NOTE

If students have challenges generating ideas on their own, make some example suggestions from the list below, then pull ideas from individuals in the group.

Tune in to any cultural differences with respect to relationships. In some communities there may be cultural beliefs about what is valued in relationships. Also, make sure you are knowledgeable about state laws regarding relationship violence and assault.

Possible answers:

- » Trust—The trust goes both ways.

- » Open communication.

- » Equality—The two people are of a similar age and have an equal say in how they spend time and make decisions. (Partners who are older and more mature tend to control what happens in the relationship because they have more experience and more resources such as money.)

- » Shared interests—They like to do many of the same things.

- » Shared values—They have similar views about what is important in life and what is right and wrong.

- » Caring, love, and affection—These feelings go both ways.

- » Respect for self and for partner.

- » They deal with conflict well—When they disagree or have arguments, they can talk things out so each person feels OK about what happened.

- » Nonviolence and emotional safety—There is no violence of any type (verbal, physical, emotional or sexual).

3. **As students offer characteristics, ask clarifying questions to help deepen their understanding of healthy relationships. For example,**

    - » How do you know when you have that thing (e.g., trust) in a relationship?

    - » What does it look like when two people trust each other?

    - » Give me some examples of open communication in a relationship.

4. **Next, ask the group what they think the signs or qualities of unhealthy relationships are. Solicit responses from the group and record their answers on the pre-labeled newsprint.**

    Possible answers:

    - » Often have miscommunication or lack of communication

    - » Controlling behavior

    - » Jealously that is extreme or frequent

    - » Differences in age, power, maturity

    - » Disrespect—name calling, put-downs, public humiliation

    - » Pressure to do things you don't want to do

    - » Being willing to do anything to hold on to a partner

 Making a Difference! For Youth with Cognitive Impairments

» Doing things you don't want to do because a partner expects it

» A partner keeping you from friends and family

» Arguments that don't get resolved often

» Stress, sadness, fear or feelings of desperation

» Engaging in behaviors that are risky to your health

» Physical, emotional or sexual abuse/violence

5. **Praise the group on the ideas they generated for the signs of healthy and unhealthy relationships.**

6. **Display the *TREO: Four Parts of Healthy Relationships* poster. Tell the group to help them remember four of the most important components of healthy relationships, you'll use the word "TREO."**

    » **Trust:** Partners trust each other and feel safe in a relationship.

    » **Respect:** First you respect yourself. Second, you respect each other.

    » **Equality:** Partners have equal amounts of power and control in the relationship.

    » **Open communication:** Partners talk openly and listen to each other.

7. **Discuss with the group how being in a healthy relationship could affect a person's ability to make proud and responsible choices about sex.**

    Be sure to make the following points:

    » A partner would care about you and want to keep you safe.

    » You would trust each other.

    » A partner would treat you like an equal and make decisions jointly instead of pressuring you or forcing you to do things.

    » You would have open communication and it would be easier to talk about sexual feelings and decisions.

8. Summarize the activity by saying,

KEY MESSAGE:

When forming relationships, look for people who can form healthy relationships with you.

Treat people in your relationships the way that you want to be treated.

Healthy relationships require trust, respect, equality and open communication.

> Now that you know the difference between healthy and unhealthy relationships, look for partners who can form a healthy relationship with you.
>
> When something happens and you get that "uh oh" feeling in your stomach… that's a warning sign of an unhealthy relationship. Pay attention.
>
> Also, relationships are a two-way street. You have to be the kind of partner that you want to have. You have to be trustworthy and communicate. You have to want to keep your partner safe.
>
> Remember TREO—trust, respect, equality and open communication are necessary for healthy relationships. It's much easier to choose proud and responsible behavior when you're in a healthy relationship.

9. Keep the filled-in newsprint with the characteristics of healthy and unhealthy relationships available for future sessions.

Making a Difference! For Youth with Cognitive Impairments

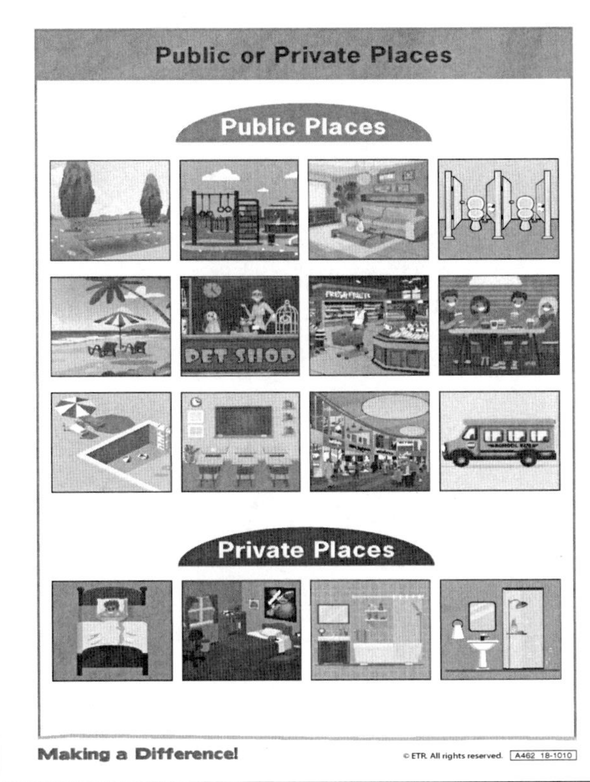

Poster

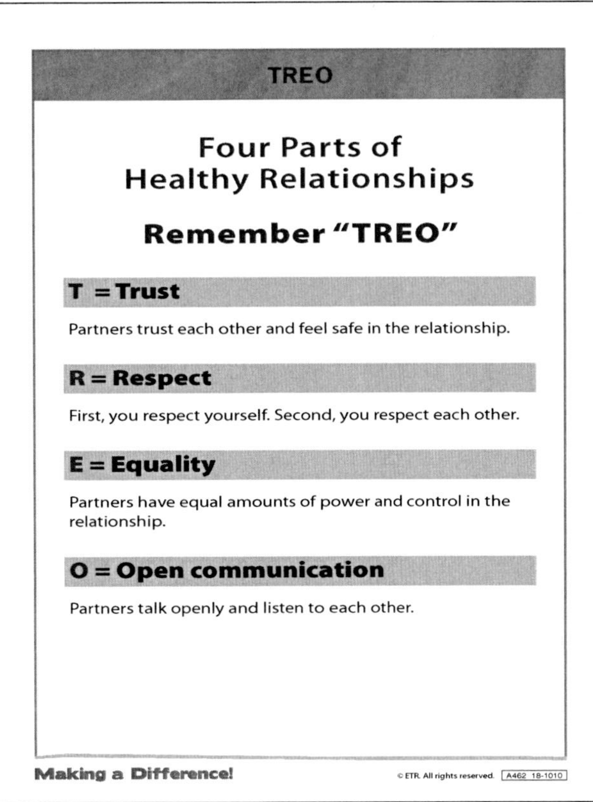

10 Cards

Poster

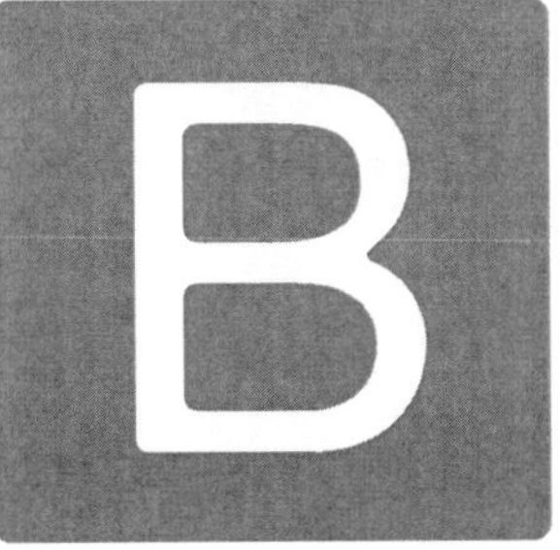

SUPPLEMENTAL BACKGROUND INFORMATION

There may be times when facilitators implementing this curriculum need some background information to help teach a given topic. This section covers supplemental background information on sexually transmitted diseases, contraceptives and the effects of alcohol and other drugs. This information is not to be taken as an in-depth review. If you need more information, please contact your Department of Health or visit the CDC website: www.cdc.gov.

Table of Contents

INFORMATION ABOUT HIV

What Is HIV?

HIV stands for human immunodeficiency virus. It is the virus that causes AIDS. People who have HIV in their bodies are said to have HIV or to be HIV-positive.

HIV damages the body's immune system, which normally protects the body from disease. In particular, HIV attacks specialized white blood cells called CD4 or T-cells. HIV takes over the machinery of the CD4 cells to make copies of itself and spread throughout the body, so the immune cells can't do their job of protecting the body. As the number of properly working T-cells decreases, the immune system becomes weaker until it can no longer fight off different types of infections.

HIV is a disease with many stages. People can live with HIV for years without getting sick. They may look and feel healthy and may not even know they have the virus. But even when a person with HIV looks and feels fine, he or she can pass the virus to others.

What is AIDS?

AIDS stands for acquired immunodeficiency syndrome. It is a condition caused by HIV. AIDS is the stage of HIV when the immune system has become very weak and damaged. When this happens, other diseases and infections can enter the body. These are called "opportunistic infections" because they take advantage of the weakened immune system.

Blood tests can be done to determine the number of CD4 cells and the amount of HIV in the blood (the viral load). The CD4 count is a standard measure of how well the immune system is working. A person with HIV is diagnosed as having AIDS when he or she has a CD4 count below 200 per cubic milliliter of blood (most people without HIV have a count of 700 to 1000) or when certain opportunistic infections occur. These may include cancers; Pneumocystis carinii, a lung infection; other viral infections; or severe weight loss.

How do people get HIV?

HIV is found in the blood, semen or vaginal fluids, and rectal fluids of someone with HIV. It is passed from person to person through these body fluids.

People can get HIV:

- **Through sex.** Anyone who has unprotected vaginal or anal sex with someone who has HIV can get HIV. There is also some risk of transmission through oral sex, but it is much lower.

 Making a Difference! For Youth with Cognitive Impairments

- **By sharing needles** for injecting drugs, vitamins, hormones or steroids. HIV-infected blood may be left in the needle or syringe and passed on to the next user. Other injection supplies (sometimes called "works") can also pass HIV (e.g., water, cotton and cookers).

- **By sharing needles** for tattooing, piercing or for any other reason.

- **From mother to child either before or during birth.** There are also a few known cases in which HIV has been passed from mother to child through breastfeeding. A pregnant woman with HIV can take medicines to greatly lower the risk of her baby being born with HIV.

As a general guideline, people should avoid having direct contact with other people's blood. This is why medical providers, including first responders, wear gloves when they are providing care that might bring them into contact with another person's blood.

Before 1985, some people got HIV from infected blood transfusions or blood products. Since 1985, the supply of blood and blood products in the United States and most developed countries has been routinely tested, making this form of transmission now extremely rare.

Ways HIV is *not* transmitted

HIV is not transmitted by casual, day-to-day contact between people. The virus is not transmitted through the air. It must get inside the body to infect a person.

People can't get HIV from:

- touching, coughing, sneezing or kissing
- toilet seats, eating utensils, swimming pools, water fountains or telephones
- casual contact such as hugging, dry kissing or sharing food
- donating blood
- tears, saliva, sweat or urine
- mosquitoes or other insects

Who is at risk for HIV?

It is what people do, not who they are, that puts them at risk for HIV.

People are at risk for HIV if:

- They have sex with someone who's had other partners.
- They have sex without using a latex condom.

- They share needles or syringes to inject drugs, or had sex with someone who has.

- They share needles or other sharp objects for tattooing, piercing or any other reason.

Babies born to women with HIV are also at risk.

People are probably not at risk if:

- They haven't ever had sex, or have had sex with only one partner, who doesn't have HIV and who's had sex only with them.

- They haven't ever shared needles to inject drugs or for any other reason, and haven't had sex with anyone who has.

How can people eliminate or reduce the risk of getting HIV?

To eliminate the risk of HIV:

- **Don't have sex.** This includes vaginal, anal and oral sex.

- **Never inject drugs, or share needles** for any reason.

To reduce the risk of HIV:

- **Use a latex condom each and every time** for vaginal, anal or oral sex. Condoms must be used consistently and correctly to ensure protection.

- **Don't use oil-based lubricants.** Oils in hand lotions, massage oils, petroleum jelly, etc., can cause a male condom to leak or break.

- **Have a monogamous relationship** with only one partner who doesn't have HIV, who doesn't use injection drugs or share needles or syringes for any reason, and who never has sex with anyone else. (*Note:* This choice isn't realistic for many teens because they tend to be involved in a series of relatively short-term relationships. It's also not a completely safe choice because some people may lie about their sexual or drug-use histories or may not know if they have HIV or another STD.)

- **Discuss HIV with a partner.** Ask about past or present risk behaviors.

- **Get tested for HIV.** Be sure any sex partner has been tested before having sex.

- **Avoid having multiple or overlapping partners.** The more sex partners a person has, the greater the chances of contracting HIV or another STD.

- **Have safer sex** that doesn't put you in contact with a partner's blood, semen or vaginal or rectal fluids. This means using condoms during vaginal or anal intercourse, using condoms or other barriers during oral sex or having sex play without intercourse.

Making a Difference! For Youth with Cognitive Impairments

- **People who use injection drugs** should never share needles. If needles or works are shared or re-used, clean them up to 3 times with water, for 30 seconds with bleach and again with water before each use.

- **Don't use alcohol, marijuana or other drugs** that impair judgment. Being high can lead to unsafe sex or other drug use.

- **If you may have been exposed to HIV** immediately contact a doctor about post-exposure prophylaxis (PEP). These medications may be able to prevent the virus from infecting the body if taken immediately after exposure (within 72 hours).

- **If a partner has HIV,** talk to a doctor about pre-exposure prophylaxis (PrEP). These medications can be taken daily to prevent HIV.

What types of HIV test are available?

The most common type of HIV test is the antibody test. The test looks for HIV antibodies in the body by testing blood or saliva. Antibodies are proteins the body makes in response to a virus. If a person has antibodies for HIV, he or she has HIV and can pass the virus to other people.

There is also an antigen test for HIV. An antigen is a protein that produces antibodies. HIV antigens can be detected very soon after infection (1–3 weeks) by testing the blood. These tests are more expensive and are not typically used for routine HIV testing. If a person has antigens for HIV, he or she has HIV and can pass the virus to other people.

The PCR *(polymerase chain reaction)* tests blood for the genetic material of HIV. Blood supplies in most developed countries are screened for HIV using PCR tests. PCR tests are also used to measure viral loads for people who are HIV-positive. If a person has HIV genetic material, he or she has HIV and can pass the virus to other people.

Tests are available at public health clinics, hospitals, state and local health departments, at community events, mobile testing vans and other locations. Many places offer free or low-cost testing. Home testing kits can be purchased at pharmacies or online.

What happens when a person gets tested?

At most HIV test sites, a counselor explains the test during a pretest session. This information may be provided one-on-one, to a couple, through a video or in a small-group session. People can ask questions and talk about their risks for HIV at this time.

Then a health worker takes a little blood from the person's arm or finger, or takes some cells from the inside of the cheek or gums with a cotton swab. It doesn't hurt and it is very quick. The sample will be sent to a lab for testing, or tested on site.

Most testing centers also help the person plan to deal with either a positive or negative result, and provide the names and phone numbers of appropriate community agencies that may be of further help (e.g., a hotline to call if the person has further questions about risk behaviors or referrals for care and treatment).

People using home kits mail a small blood or saliva sample to a lab, using a code name or number. Test results are given by telephone when the person calls and gives the code.

Where can a person go to get tested?

Easy ways to find a convenient HIV testing site include:

- calling **1-800-CDC-INFO** (232-4636)
- visiting **gettested.cdc.gov** or **locator.hiv.gov**
- texting a zip code to **KNOWIT** (566948)

Tests are available at public health clinics, hospitals, state and local health departments, community events, mobile testing vans and other locations. Many places offer free or low-cost testing. Home testing kits can be purchased at pharmacies or online. People using home kits mail a small blood or saliva sample to a lab, using a code name or number. Test results are given by telephone when the person calls and gives the code.

Can teens be tested without parent permission?

Yes, teens can consent to HIV testing without parent permission. However, to be sure, teens should check with the test site beforehand to find out what policies are followed. They can ask if they need parental consent for testing or treatment, and whether the clinic will share information with parents.

Who will know the results?

Most testing sites offer *confidential* testing. This means that the result is told only to the person taking the test, and it is also put in his or her medical file.

Some test sites offer *anonymous* testing. This means the person doesn't give a name, and the test result is reported only to him or her. Home testing kit results are anonymous.

When selecting a testing site, a person may wish to find out whether the test is anonymous or confidential, how results are verified and recorded and if before and after counseling is part of the procedure.

Making a Difference! For Youth with Cognitive Impairments

What about routine testing in clinical settings?

More than 1.1 million people in the United States are living with HIV infection, but 1 in 7 (14.2%) don't know it (CDC, 2018). They therefore can't benefit from early treatment and are likely to pass the virus to others without knowing it. To promote earlier detection and reduce stigma around testing, the Centers for Disease Control and Prevention (CDC) recommends that all patients in clinical settings be tested for HIV as part of their routine medical care unless the person opts out. HIV screening should also be included in the routine panel of prenatal tests for all pregnant women. People at high risk of HIV infection should get tested at least once a year. In 2012, Congress passed a law (H.R. 4470 Routine HIV Screening Coverage Act of 2012) requiring health insurance to cover the cost of these screenings.

In health care settings, pretest prevention counseling and informed consent are not required in order to reduce barriers to testing in these settings. CDC believes HIV testing can be covered under a general permission form (consent form) that is signed for all medical care.

How long does it take to get the results?

Laboratory test results can take up to 2 weeks. Many clinics now offer a rapid test, with results available within 30 minutes. If the rapid test is positive, the sample needs to be tested again to be sure. Results of the confirmation test can take up to 2 weeks.

Home testing kit results take around 7 days, or as little as 3 days if mailed using an overnight mail service.

What does it mean if the test result is positive?

A series of tests are performed on positive samples. A confirmed positive test means antibodies, antigens or HIV genetic material were found in the body. The person is then known to have HIV.

Most sites provide counseling for people testing positive. The counselor will help people deal with the stress and emotional issues, discuss what to do to maintain health, and explain how to prevent transmitting HIV to others.

What does it mean if the test result is negative?

If the initial test result is negative, it means no antibodies to HIV were found in the person's blood. No further testing is called for, and most likely the person tested is not infected.

However, a person who was exposed to HIV recently (generally within 3 months or, in rare instances, up to 6 months before testing) may not yet have developed antibodies that can be detected by the test. If a person has tested negative on the HIV antibody test but has had some HIV-related risk within the past 6 months, it's important for that person to stop the risky behavior and be tested again 6 months after the last risky behavior to be sure of the results.

How long does it take for an HIV test to show that a person has HIV?

The "window period" is the length of time between when a person first gets HIV and when an HIV test can begin to detect signs of the virus in the body. It can be from 2 weeks to 3 months long, depending on the type of test that is done. During the window period, even before they know they are infected, people can transmit HIV to others.

Are there treatments for HIV?

Yes. The sooner people find out they have HIV, the earlier they can begin getting care and treatment. An early diagnosis allows people to participate in decisions about their treatment and begin taking medicines to strengthen the immune system and decrease the amount of the virus in the body.

There is no cure for HIV, but anti-retroviral treatments (ART) can be started while the person still feels healthy. With ART medicines, people with HIV can lead longer and healthier lives than ever before. The most common treatments limit the ability of the virus to reproduce. They help protect the immune system and improve the chances of staying healthy.

Pregnant women with HIV can take medicines to greatly reduce the baby's risk of having HIV.

Will everyone with HIV get sick eventually?

While complications from HIV infection are possible, current treatments and medications are giving people with HIV a positive prognosis and near-normal life-span. If people with HIV remain in medical care and are able to continue to take the medications to keep low viral loads, they can live long, healthy lives. Patients living with HIV would then be vulnerable to the same health conditions that affect all people as they age.

 Making a Difference! For Youth with Cognitive Impairments

How is HIV treated?

HIV treatment consists of the ongoing, monitored use of a drug or drugs. Treatment has
3 main goals:

- Some medications slow the spread of HIV. Different types of these antiviral drugs
  interfere at different stages in the production of HIV by the body. Using several
  antiviral drugs together in combination treatment has been found to slow the
  progress of HIV significantly.

- Some medicines make the immune system stronger.

- Other medicines prevent or treat opportunistic infections. These drugs can slow or
  stop many of the diseases, cancers or illnesses a person with HIV can get when the
  immune system has become very weak.

There are different "classes" of HIV drugs that work in different ways to stop the virus from
replicating in the body. Each class of drug attacks the virus at different points in its life
cycle. Typically, people are prescribed a combination of 3 different HIV medicines to control
the amount of virus in the body and protect the immune system. The combination of
medicines also helps prevent HIV drug resistance.

When deciding about treatment, the person with HIV and his or her health care provider
consider how healthy the person feels, the viral load, the person's ability to take the
medicines as directed, current life circumstances, and how the treatment may affect the
person's health in the future. There may be social and environmental factors that affect
a person's ability to remain in medical care and to continue taking HIV medicines. When
people begin treatment for HIV, they may need other services and support to stay healthy
(for example housing, mental health care, food assistance, support groups and medication
management programs).

It's important for people with HIV to work closely with an HIV treatment team to identify the
most appropriate treatment plan to meet their needs and support long-term health and
wellness.

SEXUALLY TRANSMITTED DISEASES (STD)

WHAT IS AN STD?

Sexually transmitted disease (STD) is a term used to categorize a group of infections typically transmitted through vaginal, oral or anal sex. You may also hear the term STI or sexually transmitted infection. Most STDs are caused by either bacteria or viruses. Typically STDs caused by bacteria can be cured and those caused by viruses cannot be cured. However, all types can be treated and prevented.

TYPES OF STDs

CHLAMYDIA

Organism: Caused by a **bacterium** called *Chlamydia trachomatis*

How Transmitted: Vaginal, anal and oral sex

Symptoms: **Females** – Thick yellow vaginal discharge, irregular periods, bleeding with intercourse and/or burning and pain during urination

Males – Watery white discharge from penis and burning and/or pain during urination

However, most people with chlamydia do not have any symptoms.

Complications: **Females** – If left untreated, can cause pelvic inflammatory disease (PID), tubal pregnancy and infertility. **About 10–15% of women with untreated chlamydia get pelvic inflammatory disease (PID).** A pregnant woman with chlamydia can also give the infection to her fetus, which can cause premature birth, miscarriage or intrauterine death. In newborns, it can also cause low birth weight, pneumonia and/or conjunctivitis (an eye infection).

Males – If left untreated, infection can spread from the urethra (area responsible for urination/pee) to the testicles, causing swelling, tenderness and even sterility. It can also lead to a more widespread infection that includes conjunctivitis (eye infection), arthritis and skin lesions.

Making a Difference! For Youth with Cognitive Impairments

Having chlamydia increases the risk of being infected with HIV if exposed, and of passing HIV to a partner if HIV positive.

Diagnosis: Must have a test to know you are infected. The CDC recommends annual screening for sexually active women age 25 and younger. Gay, bisexual and other men who have sex with men, as well as pregnant women, should also get tested for chlamydia.

Treatment: Easily treated with antibiotics. A person with chlamydia is also tested for gonorrhea since these infections can coexist. The partner(s) of the infected person must also be treated. Once treated, a person is cured. However, a person can be reinfected if exposed to chlamydia again.

SYPHILIS

Organism: Caused by a **bacterium** called *Treponema pallidum*

How Transmitted: Direct contact with sores through vaginal, anal or oral sex or touching

Symptoms: **Females and Males** – Symptoms begin 1–12 weeks after infection and occur in three stages.

First Stage – Symptoms include the appearance of a sore called a chancre and swelling of the lymph nodes near the groin. The sore usually is small, round and painless. It lasts 3–6 weeks and heals on its own regardless of whether the person gets treated. But, if untreated, the infection progresses to the second stage. There may be multiple sores.

Second Stage – The second stage of syphilis begins as the sore heals or several weeks after it heals. Symptoms include the appearance of a red, bumpy, scaly, non-itchy rash. The rash may come and go and includes spots on the palms of the hands and soles of the feet. On the face, the rash may look like acne. Slimy white patches in the mouth or on the genitals, wart-like growths around the anus, patchy hair loss and flu-like symptoms (headache, fever, body aches, fatigue, loss of appetite) may also occur. This stage lasts from weeks to a year.

Latent Stage – After the second stage, most people who are untreated enter the latent stage. This stage has no symptoms and may last a lifetime.

Third Stage – About 15% of untreated people who enter the latent stage of syphilis go on to develop tertiary syphilis—the third stage of infection. This begins 10–30 years after the initial infection. It can cause heart disease, brain damage, paralysis, blindness and even death.

Complications: Damage to the body that occurs prior to treatment may not be reversible.

A woman can give the disease to her fetus during pregnancy or have a miscarriage. Babies infected with syphilis are often born prematurely and can develop problems with their eyes, central nervous systems, bones, liver and spleen. They may also have swollen lymph nodes, yellow skin (jaundice), skin rash and anemia.

Having syphilis increases the risk of being infected with HIV if exposed, and of passing HIV to a partner if HIV positive.

Diagnosis: Must be tested to know if you have the infection.

Treatment: Easily treated with penicillin and other antibiotics.

- -

GONORRHEA

Organism: Caused by a **bacterium** called *Neisseria gonorrhoeae*

How Transmitted: Direct contact with infected person through vaginal, anal or oral sex

Symptoms: **Females –** Burning and pain during urination, frequent urination, thick yellow discharge. Mild symptoms can be mistaken for a bladder or vaginal infection.

Most women with gonorrhea do not have any symptoms.

Males – Burning and/or pain during urination, discharge from penis.

Some men with gonorrhea have no symptoms at all.

Rectal Gonorrhea – Can result from anal sex. Symptoms such as rectal discharge and discomfort around anus can occur, but infection is usually asymptomatic.

Gonococcal Pharyngitis – Can result from oral sex. Symptoms include sore throat, difficulty swallowing and red, swollen tonsils.

Complications: **Females –** If left untreated, infection can lead to pelvic inflammatory disease (PID), ectopic pregnancy and infertility. Can also lead to more widespread infection that includes arthritis and skin lesions on the arms and legs. A pregnant woman can give the infection to her baby during childbirth. This can cause serious health problems for the baby.

Males – If left untreated, infection can spread from the urethra to the testicles and cause sterility. Can also lead to a more widespread infection that includes arthritis and skin lesions.

Having gonorrhea increases the risk of being infected with HIV if exposed, and of passing HIV to a partner if HIV positive.

Diagnosis: Must be tested to know if you have the infection.

Treatment: Can be treated with antibiotics. A person diagnosed with gonorrhea is also tested for chlamydia since these infections often coexist. The partner(s) of the infected person must also be tested. Once treated, a person is cured. However, a person can be reinfected if exposed to gonorrhea again.

HERPES

Organism: Caused by a **virus** called *herpes simplex virus (HSV)*. There are two types:

- HSV Type 1: Usually causes cold sores or fever blisters; can be spread from mouth to genitals during oral sex
- HSV Type 2: Can cause sores/blisters on the genitals

Either type 1 or type 2 can cause a herpes infection in the mouth, eyes, vagina, penis or anal area.

How Transmitted: Direct contact with infected person through vaginal, anal or oral sex, kissing, or skin-to-skin contact

A person with herpes can infect someone else just by "rubbing" when they have a sore; for example, rubbing the penis against the vulva without having clothes on. **THIS MEANS YOU DO NOT HAVE TO HAVE SEXUAL INTERCOURSE TO GET HERPES.**

The easiest way to pass herpes is through contact with the sores. HOWEVER, a person infected with herpes does not have to have sores to pass the virus/infection on to someone else. Women can also pass this infection to a baby during childbirth.

Symptoms: **Females and Males –** Painful sores on the vagina, penis, anal area or mouth. These sores tend to recur. This means that even if herpes sores go away, they often come back. This may happen for the rest of a person's life. **Some people do not have any symptoms.**

Complications: Women can pass the infection to their babies during childbirth.

Having herpes increases the risk of being infected with HIV if exposed, and of passing HIV to a partner if HIV positive.

Diagnosis: Must have a test to know if you are infected. The doctor swabs a small amount from the sore and tests the cells to see if it contains the virus.

Treatment: **There is no cure for herpes,** only treatment for the symptoms (sores). Most patients are treated with Acyclovir (Zovirax) to slow down the recurrence of the sores and ease the pain during an outbreak. Since sores come back when a person is under stress, it is also recommended that an infected person get plenty of rest, stay away from stressful situations, exercise and eat healthy.

HPV

Organism: Caused by *human papillomavirus,* a **virus** with more than 100 types

How Transmitted: Direct contact with infected person through vaginal, anal or oral sex, or skin-to-skin contact

A person with HPV can infect someone else just by "rubbing," for example, rubbing the penis against the vulva without having clothes on. **THIS MEANS YOU DO NOT HAVE TO HAVE SEXUAL INTERCOURSE TO GET HPV.**

Making a Difference! For Youth with Cognitive Impairments

Symptoms: **Females and Males** – Soft, moist, pink, fleshy warts that can look like cauliflower. They are usually painless and can be raised, pointed or flat in shape. Usually they appear in clusters, but they can also grow alone. If left untreated, warts may go away, stay the same or grow and spread. Most people do not have any symptoms.

Complications: Women can pass this infection to their babies during childbirth.

Most people with HPV do not develop health problems from it, but some types of the virus can cause genital warts, and others can lead to cervical cancer or cancer of the vulva, vagina, penis, anus or back of the throat.

Diagnosis: Genital warts can usually be diagnosed by physical exam or their appearance. An HPV test can screen for cervical cancer.

Treatment: Warts can be treated with a chemical cream or they can be removed. A doctor will determine the best course of treatment. However, because HPV may be a lifelong infection, treatment may clear only the warts and not the infection.

Prevention: Vaccines can protect males and females against some of the most common types of HPV that cause problems. The number of vaccines can vary. It is important to get all doses to get the best protection. The vaccines are most effective when given before a person's first sexual contact, prior to possible exposure to HPV.

Females – Vaccines are available to protect females against the types of HPV that cause most cervical cancers. Two of these vaccines also protect against most genital warts.

Males – Two vaccines protect males against most genital warts and some kinds of HPV-related cancer.

TRICHOMONIASIS

Organism: Caused by a **single-cell protozoan parasite** called *Trichomonas vaginalis*

How Transmitted: Direct contact with infected person through vaginal sex

Symptoms: **Females** – Frothy, yellow-green vaginal discharge with a strong

Appendix B // SUPPLEMENTAL BACKGROUND INFORMATION

odor. May also cause discomfort during sexual intercourse and urination, as well as irritation and itching of the genitals. Sometimes, lower abdominal pain can occur.

Males – Most men with trichomoniasis do not have signs or symptoms; however, some men may temporarily have an irritation inside the penis, mild discharge or slight burning after urination or ejaculation.

Complications:

Pregnant women with trichomoniasis may have babies who are born early or with low birth weight.

If left untreated, the genital inflammation caused by trichomoniasis can increase the risk of being infected with HIV if exposed, and of passing HIV to a partner if HIV positive.

Diagnosis:

Must be tested to know if you have the infection.

Treatment:

Trichomoniasis can be treated and cured with prescription drugs, either metronidazole or tinidazole, given by mouth in a single dose. The partner(s) of the person infected must also be tested and treated. Once treated, a person is cured. However, a person can be reinfected if exposed to trichomoniasis again.

HEPATITIS B

Organism:

Caused by a **virus** called *hepatitis B virus (HBV)*

How Transmitted:

Hepatitis B is transmitted through activities that involve percutaneous (i.e., puncture through the skin) or mucosal contact with infectious blood or body fluids (e.g., semen, saliva).

Symptoms:

Symptoms begin an average of 90 days (or 3 months) after exposure to the virus, but they can appear any time between 8 weeks and 5 months after exposure. Symptoms can include fever, fatigue, loss of appetite, nausea, vomiting, abdominal pain, dark urine, clay-colored bowel movements, joint pain and jaundice.

Complications:

Hepatitis B can develop from an acute (short-lived) infection into a chronic infection that leads to a disease of the liver that can be very serious. Liver damage in chronic hepatitis B, if not stopped, continues until the liver becomes hardened and scarlike. This is called cirrhosis, a condition traditionally associated with alcoholism.

Making a Difference! For Youth with Cognitive Impairments

When this happens, the liver can no longer carry out its normal
functions, a condition called liver failure. The only treatment for
liver failure is liver transplant.

Diagnosis: Must be tested to know if you have the infection.

Treatment: If a healthcare provider determines the hepatitis B infection is acute
(short-lived), the person may not need treatment. Instead, the
healthcare provider will work to reduce any signs and symptoms
experienced while the person's body fights the infection. If the
case is chronic, the healthcare provider may recommend antiviral
medications, or in severe cases, liver transplant.

Prevention: There is a vaccine that can prevent hepatitis B. It is recommended
for infants, people age 18 and younger who were not vaccinated as
infants, and adults who are at risk.

HIV

Organism: Caused by a **virus** called *human immunodeficiency virus* that
damages a person's body by destroying specific blood cells, called
CD4 cells, or T cells, which are crucial to helping the body fight
diseases.

How Transmitted: HIV is primarily spread by unprotected anal or vaginal sex. It can
also be spread by oral sex, sharing needles or syringes, or from a
mother to her fetus.

Symptoms: The only way to know if you are infected is to be tested for HIV.
People cannot rely on symptoms to know whether or not they are
infected. However, the following may be warning signs of advanced
HIV infection: rapid weight loss; dry cough; recurring fever or
profuse night sweats; profound and unexplained fatigue; swollen
lymph glands in the armpits, groin or neck; diarrhea that lasts for
more than a week; white spots or unusual blemishes on the tongue,
in the mouth or in the throat; pneumonia; red, brown, pink or
purplish blotches on or under the skin or inside the mouth, nose or
eyelids; memory loss; depression; and other neurological disorders.

Complications:	HIV infection, if left untreated with anti-retroviral drugs, can lead to AIDS (acquired immunodeficiency syndrome). HIV infection weakens the immune system, making an infected person highly susceptible to a number of bacterial, viral, fungal and parasitic infections. It can also make an infected person more susceptible to certain types of cancers.
	Infections can include pneumonia, tuberculosis, viral hepatitis, herpes simplex virus, human papillomavirus, meningitis and non-Hodgkin's lymphoma.
Diagnosis:	Must be tested to know if you have the infection.
Treatment:	There is no cure for HIV; however, there are treatment options that can help people living with HIV experience long and productive lives. Anti-retroviral medications inhibit the growth and replication of HIV at various stages of its life cycle. There are several classes of these drugs available, and the options should be discussed with a healthcare provider.
Prevention:	Post-exposure prophylaxis (PEP) is treatment with medicines that may be able to prevent the virus from infecting the body if taken within 72 hours of exposure. Pre-exposure prophylaxis (PrEP) involves taking daily medication to lower the chances of infection. It is most often used by people with HIV-positive partners or others at high risk.

HOW TO PREVENT AN STD

The most effective way to prevent an STD is to *NOT HAVE SEX*, either oral, anal or vaginal. People who choose to have sex need to use a latex or polyurethane/polyisoprene condom each time.

Remember:

- You cannot tell by just looking if someone has an STD.
- For some of the most common STDs (chlamydia, gonorrhea, HPV), many people never have any symptoms.

Making a Difference! For Youth with Cognitive Impairments

- Some people with STDs never get treated because they did not have symptoms or the symptoms disappeared. These people were never cured and may have passed the infection to others.

- Washing, urinating or douching does not prevent STDs.

- You can get an STD again and again.

- You can get an STD if you have sex only once.

- Once you are infected with a viral STD such as herpes you are always infected— there is no cure.

WHAT TO DO IF YOU THINK YOU HAVE AN STD

See a health provider. If you have been sexually active, have not used condoms and know or think your sex partner has an STD you need to ask the doctor to test you, even if you have no symptoms. The tests are simple and are the only way to know for sure if you are infected with an STD.

Remember:

- Always use a latex or polyurethane/polyisoprene condom.

- If you or your partner(s) have unusual discharge, sores or rashes on or near the vagina, penis or anal area, STOP having sex, get tested and get treated if needed.

- If you have an STD, TAKE ALL YOUR MEDICINE EVEN IF YOU FEEL BETTER OR THE SYMPTOMS GO AWAY.

- Tell your partner(s) that you have an STD and that they should be tested and treated. If your partner(s) do not get treated and you continue to have sex, you may be reinfected. BE RESPONSIBLE!

CONTRACEPTIVE METHODS

Condoms are only one of many birth control methods that exist. However, **they are the only method besides abstinence that can effectively prevent the transmission of sexually transmitted infections, including HIV.** The other methods of protection described here are effective only in preventing pregnancy.

Adolescents can obtain two types of contraceptive methods: prescribed methods that must be obtained from a health care provider, or over-the-counter methods that can be purchased from a store without a prescription. Contraceptives can also be categorized as hormonal methods (e.g., birth control pills and Depo-Provera) and barrier methods (e.g., condoms and diaphragms). Except for abstinence and condoms, use of any of the following methods should be coupled with consistent condom usage for STD prevention.

This section describes the methods in order of effectiveness.

Abstinence (Choosing Not to Have Sex)

What it is: Not engaging in sexual activities; also called abstinence. Choosing not to have sex means refraining from any sexual activity that can result in pregnancy and STDs, including vaginal, oral and anal sex, as well as skin-to-skin genital contact that can transmit certain STDs.

How it works: Individuals or couples decide that not having sex (vaginal, anal and/or oral) is the best decision for them. People decide to do this for many reasons. They find other ways of showing their love and affection. They learn ways to tell their partners how they feel so they can stick with their decision.

How to use it: Choosing not to have sex is the simplest of all methods to use. It's free. You don't have to store it in a special place.

How and where to get it: You've got it. It's free.

Effectiveness and advantages: Choosing not to have sex is the safest and most effective method of preventing HIV, other STD and pregnancy. It works all the time when people consistently avoid any behaviors that can potentially result in pregnancy or STD.

Risks and disadvantages: There are no health risks. People need to be prepared to deal with pressure if a partner doesn't agree that abstinence is the best choice.

Making a Difference! For Youth with Cognitive Impairments

Long-Acting Reversible Contraception (LARC)

IUD

What it is: The IUD (intrauterine device) is a small, plastic device shaped like a "T" that is inserted into the uterus by a doctor. There are five IUDs currently on the market—the Copper T, Mirena, Skyla, Liletta and Kyleena. Depending on the type of IUD, it can provide protection from pregnancy for 3 to 10 years. IUDs are reversible, meaning they can be removed by a health care provider and do not have to stay in place for a set number of years.

How it works: The IUD prevents pregnancy by affecting the way sperm move and preventing sperm from fertilizing an egg. Some IUDs (Mirena, Skyla) also release hormones that prevent pregnancy the same way as the birth control pill.

How to use it: The IUD must be inserted by a health care provider. After it is inserted, no further action for pregnancy prevention is required. The IUD is an approved method for young women, including teens (American College of Obstetricians and Gynecologists, 2012).

How and where to get it: IUDs must be obtained from a health care provider. The provider puts the IUD into the uterus through the vagina, using a small tube. The sides of the "T" collapse into a skinny straight line when it goes into the body, so it doesn't poke the vagina or uterus. The procedure can be done at the clinic or doctor's office.

Effectiveness and advantages: The IUD is highly effective (more than 99%) at preventing pregnancy. IUDs wrapped with copper (Copper T) provide protection for up to 10 years. Hormonal IUDs (Skyla, Liletta, Mirena, Kyleena) provide protection for 3 to 5 years. Some people prefer to use an IUD because it is very private and always in place and they don't have to remember to take a pill each day. It can be removed by a health care provider at any time, and fertility rapidly returns to previous levels after removal.

Risks and disadvantages: *The IUD doesn't protect against HIV or other STD.* Side effects may include changes to the menstrual cycle, more bleeding and cramping during periods or spotting between periods. It must be inserted and removed by a health care provider.

Implant

What it is: The implant is a single thin rod or tube of artificial hormones (progestin) placed under the skin of the upper arm by a health care provider. Implants work for at least 3 years and are reversible, meaning they can be removed by a health care provider at the end of their period of efficacy or earlier if women want to get pregnant or change methods.

How it works: The implant slowly releases a low dose of the hormone progestin into the bloodstream. This stops the ovaries from releasing eggs. It also thickens cervical mucus, which makes it more difficult for sperm to reach the egg.

How to use it: Implants must be inserted by a health care provider. After insertion, no further action for pregnancy prevention is required until the 3-year period expires. The implant is an approved method for young women, including teens (American College of Obstetricians and Gynecologists, 2012).

How and where to get it: Implants must be obtained from a health care provider. A small incision is made on the inside of the upper arm; then the rod, which is about the size of a matchstick, is inserted. The procedure can be done at the clinic or doctor's office with a local anesthetic.

Effectiveness and advantages: The implant is highly effective (more than 99%) at preventing pregnancy, and it provides protection for 3 years. Some people prefer to use it because it is very private and always in place and they don't have to remember to take a pill each day. It can be removed by a health care provider at any time, and fertility rapidly returns to previous levels after removal.

Risks and disadvantages: *The implant doesn't protect against HIV or other STD.* Side effects may include spotting between periods, light periods, longer periods or no periods at all. It must be inserted and removed by a health care provider.

Hormonal Methods

Depo-Provera®

What it is: Depo-Provera® is an injectable form of birth control that uses a synthetic hormone (progestin) to prevent pregnancy.

How it works: Depo-Provera® injections inhibit ovulation by suppressing hormone levels. Depo-Provera® also inhibits the development of the endometrium (the lining of the uterus) and contributes to the development of thick cervical mucus that decreases sperm penetration.

How to use it: Depo-Provera® must be obtained from a health care provider. For immediate protection, the first shot needs to be received during the first 5 days of a normal menstrual period; but an additional form of contraception should be used for 2 weeks after the first

Making a Difference! For Youth with Cognitive Impairments

injection as a precautionary measure. After that, no further action is needed. Depo-Provera® provides protection all day, every day—*as long as people return to the doctor's office every 12 weeks for an injection.*

How and where to get it: Depo-Provera® requires a prescription from a doctor. People must visit their doctors every 12 weeks to receive an injection. According to the manufacturer, Depo-Provera® costs about the same per year as birth control pills.

Effectiveness and advantages: Depo-Provera® is extremely effective at preventing pregnancy (more than 99%), as long as the injections are done on schedule. Other than receiving an injection every 12 weeks, no other steps are required for protection against pregnancy. Some people prefer to use Depo-Provera® because it is very private and they don't have to remember to take a pill each day.

Risks and disadvantages: Like the pill, ***Depo-Provera® doesn't protect against HIV or other STD.*** There are several potential side effects, including weight gain and irregular or unpredictable menstrual bleeding. Other side effects may include nervousness, dizziness, stomach discomfort, headaches, fatigue or a decrease in the amount of mineral stored in the bones (a possible risk-factor for osteoporosis).

People should talk with their health care providers to ensure that Depo-Provera® is a good option for them, and must visit the doctor every 12 weeks for the injections. Once the injections are stopped, fertility will not return for an average of 6 months to 1 year. However, this period of potential "infertility" should not be regarded as a "safe" time to have unprotected intercourse.

Birth Control Pill

What it is: The birth control pill is a prescription drug that contains different amounts of the hormones estrogen and progesterone.

How it works: The pill mimics the hormones of pregnancy. It stops the release of fertile eggs from the ovaries, and thickens the mucus in the cervix so it is hard for sperm to enter the uterus.

How to use it: Birth control pills must be obtained from a health care provider. The person takes 1 pill at approximately the same time each day, as prescribed. After finishing the first pack of pills she is protected all day, every day—*as long as she continues to take the pills as prescribed.*

How and where to get it: The person must make an appointment with a health care provider, who will provide the pills at that time or write a prescription for the birth control pills with instructions about when to begin taking them.

Effectiveness and advantages: The birth control pill is more than 99% effective at preventing pregnancy if the person takes it every day, uses some other method of protection during the first month and doesn't use another person's pills. The pill is convenient and does not affect the spontaneity of a sexual relationship.

While a person taking the pill, periods may be lighter, shorter and more regular, with less cramping. The pill may protect from other health care issues, such as pelvic inflammatory disease and ovarian and endometrial cancer.

Risks and disadvantages: *The birth control pill doesn't protect against HIV or other STD.* There may be several minor side effects, including nausea, sore breasts, weight gain, skin problems and depression. A health care provider will discuss rare health risks, such as high blood pressure, blood clots, heart attack and stroke, especially for those who smoke.

Birth Control Patch & Vaginal Ring

What they are: The birth control patch is a thin plastic square that can be worn on the skin of the buttocks, stomach, upper outer arm or upper torso (but not on the breasts). The vaginal ring is a soft, flexible ring inserted into the vagina.

How they work: The patch or ring slowly releases artificial hormones into the body. They prevent pregnancy in the same ways as the birth control pill, by stopping the release of fertile eggs from the ovaries, and thickening the mucus in the cervix so it is hard for sperm to enter the uterus.

How to use them: The patch or the ring must be obtained from a health care provider. They are worn every day. A new patch is applied each week. The ring is changed once a month.

How and where to get them: The patch and the ring must be prescribed by a health care provider. People can place the patch on the body or insert the ring themselves, but must see a health care provider to get them.

Effectiveness and advantages: The patch and the ring are more than 99% effective in preventing pregnancy when they are used correctly. This means remembering to wear the patch and change it each week or to insert the ring and change it each month. The patch and the ring are simple and easy to use, as long as they are worn and changed as required.

For many, these methods are convenient and don't interfere with the spontaneity of a sexual relationship. The patch and the ring can lessen the bleeding and cramping of heavy or painful menstrual periods.

 Making a Difference! For Youth with Cognitive Impairments

Risks and disadvantages: *The patch and the ring don't protect against HIV or other STD.* They must be worn every day, whether people are having sex or not. A health care provider will discuss rare health risks, such as high blood pressure, blood clots, heart attack and stroke, especially for those who smoke.

Barrier Methods

Male Condom (External Condoms)

What it is: A male latex condom is a sheath made of thin latex rubber that fits over an erect penis. Condoms are also called "rubbers" or "prophylactics." There are alternatives for people allergic or sensitive to latex, including polyurethane (a type of plastic) and polyisoprene (a non-latex rubber).

How it works: The condom fits snugly over the erect penis and catches semen and sperm when the man ejaculates. Condoms provide a mechanical barrier that prevents direct contact with semen, sperm and other body fluids that can contain sexually transmitted bacteria and viruses, including HIV.

A common misperception is that condoms contain "holes," and that HIV can pass through the holes. Laboratory studies show that intact *latex, polyurethane* or *polyisoprene* condoms provide a continuous barrier to microorganisms, including HIV.

How to use it: The condom is unrolled onto the erect penis before the penis is placed anywhere near the partner's body.

Air pollution, heat and sunlight can weaken latex condoms. Leaving condoms in sunlight for 8–10 hours begins to weaken their strength. Condoms should not be stored for long periods in a wallet, pants pocket or glove compartment of a car. They can probably be kept safely in a wallet for up to a month. Condoms should be stored in a cool, dry place, and the package should not be opened until the condom is to be used. A condom can be used only once, and should not be used after the expiration date on the package or if it is visibly damaged.

Oil-based lubricants such as petroleum jelly, hand lotions, baby oil or other oils can weaken latex condoms and should not be used. Lubricants should be water-based, such as K-Y Jelly®, Glide®, surgical jellies and most contraceptive jellies.

How and where to get it: Condoms are available at markets, drugstores, family planning and STD clinics and online. They also may be available in vending machines or at schools. Anyone can buy condoms, regardless of age or gender. No prescription is needed.

Effectiveness and advantages: Latex condoms can be 98% effective in preventing pregnancy, but only if they are used correctly and consistently (i.e., *every time* a person has sex); this represents *perfect use*. Several studies of "discordant couples" (couples in which one member is infected with HIV and the other is not) show that using latex condoms with every act of intercourse also substantially reduces the risk of HIV transmission.

Condoms are double-dipped in latex during the manufacturing process (latex gloves are only single-dipped). Condoms are regulated by the FDA, and are subject to stringent testing. Condoms are relatively easy to use. With practice, they can become a regular, pleasurable part of a sexual relationship.

Risks and disadvantages: Condom effectiveness depends on how the condom is used. Studies have found that most latex condom failure results from user errors, such as using the condom incorrectly (e.g., using after genital contact, failing to unroll the condom completely, using oil-based lubricants), using the condom inconsistently or using a damaged condom (e.g., a condom that has been torn by fingernails or jewelry, or that has been stored improperly). ***In terms of pregnancy prevention, first year failure rates among typical users average about 18%.***

There are no serious health risks. Sometimes condoms may irritate the skin, especially if they contain a spermicide or if the user is allergic to latex. Use of another brand or a hypoallergenic (polyurethane or polyisoprene) condom will solve this problem in most cases. Use of condoms lubricated with the spermicide called nonoxynol-9 is no longer recommended. Some couples complain that condoms reduce sexual feelings. Others say it makes no difference. Some people complain about having to stop and put on the condom; but if the couple puts it on together, it can become a part of their shared responsibility within the relationship.

Natural membrane (also known as lambskin) condoms will not protect from HIV and other STD to the same degree as latex condoms.

Making a Difference! For Youth with Cognitive Impairments

Female Condom (Insertive Condoms)

What it is: The female or insertive condom is a thin, loose-fitting polyurethane or nitrile pouch that contains a flexible ring at each end. One ring lies inside the closed end of the pouch and is used to insert the condom into the vagina; it also holds the condom in place. The other ring forms the open edge of the pouch and remains outside the body after the condom is inserted.

How it works: Condoms provide a physical barrier that prevents direct contact with semen, sperm and other body fluids that can sexually transmit bacteria and viruses, including HIV.

How to use it: A person inserts the end of the condom with the ring inside into the vagina. The outside ring should lie on the vulva outside of the body. ***Female condoms should* not *be used along with male condoms.*** If both types of condoms are used at the same time, neither will stay in place. A condom can be used only once, and should not be used after the expiration date. It can be inserted up to 8 hours before intercourse, but most people insert it between 2 and 20 minutes before having sex. The condom should be removed after intercourse and thrown away in the trash.

How and where to get it: Female condoms may be purchased at drugstores or online without a prescription and are sometimes available at family planning or STD health centers. Anyone can buy condoms, regardless of age or gender.

Effectiveness and advantages: When used correctly and consistently, the female condom can be 95% effective in preventing pregnancy, and also provides protection from HIV and other STD. It offers a barrier contraceptive option that can be used instead of a male condom. It can be obtained without a prescription. If it is inserted early, it does not interrupt sex. The nitrile used in the condom is stronger than latex, has good heat-transfer characteristics that can increase pleasure, is not susceptible to deterioration with oil-based products and is less susceptible than latex to deterioration during storage.

Risks and disadvantages: Consistent and correct use is essential for effectiveness with the female condom. There are no serious health risks; however, some have reported minor issues using the condom. It may be awkward to insert without practice. A couple must be aware of keeping the condom in place as it can be pushed inside the body during sex, or the penis can slip to the side of the condom. Other problems may include minor irritation, discomfort and breakage.

Vaginal Barriers

Diaphragm, Cervical Cap, Sponge

What they are: Vaginal barriers are devices that cover the cervix (opening to the uterus) to keep sperm from reaching and fertilizing an egg. They come in different forms.

- The diaphragm is a reusable flexible, dome-shaped cup made of latex or silicone. It is inserted in the vagina and positioned to cover the cervix. It can be inserted up to 6 hours before sex, and must be left in place at least 6 but no more than 24 hours after intercourse.

- The cervical cap is a reusable silicone cap that fits over the cervix. It provides protection for 48 hours. Like the diaphragm it is inserted in the vagina before sex, and must be left in place for 6 hours after intercourse.

- The sponge is made of soft polyurethane that contains spermicide. It is inserted in the vagina before intercourse and provides protection for 24 hours. It, too, must be left in place for at least 6 hours after intercourse, but should not be left in the vagina for any more than 30 hours total. The sponge is not reusable.

How they work: Vaginal barriers prevent fertilization by blocking sperm from entering the uterus and fallopian tubes, so the sperm cannot reach the egg.

How to use them: Vaginal barriers are inserted into the vagina to cover the cervix before intercourse. The diaphragm and cervical cap should be coated with spermicide before insertion. The sponge should be moistened with water and has spermicide built in.

How and where to get them: A person must be fitted for a diaphragm or cervical cap by a health care provider. The sponge comes in one size and is available at drugstores, family planning clinics and some supermarkets.

Effectiveness and advantages: If used correctly with spermicide every time a couple has sexual intercourse, vaginal barriers are fairly effective at preventing pregnancy (diaphragm, 88–94%; sponge, 76–91%; cervical cap, 71–86%); the range in effectiveness reflects *typical use* (not always using the method consistently and correctly) versus *perfect use* (always using the method consistently and correctly). The sponge and cervical cap are more effective for those who have not had children. When used *with a latex or polyurethane condom,* the combined method is very effective at preventing pregnancy, HIV and other STD. If they are inserted early, use does not require an interruption in lovemaking. The diaphragm and cervical cap are reusable.

Making a Difference! For Youth with Cognitive Impairments

Risks and disadvantages: There are no health risks associated with using vaginal barriers. Some people may have an allergic reaction to the material the barrier is made of or the spermicide used with it. There is a low risk of vaginal or urinary infections. To avoid a very low risk of toxic shock syndrome, people should not leave a vaginal barrier method in the body longer than recommended. ***When used alone, vaginal barriers with spermicides do not protect from HIV and other STD.***

Vaginal Spermicides

Contraceptive Foam, Gel, Cream, Film, Suppositories or Tablets

What they are: Spermicides are made up of 2 components: a base or carrier (i.e., foam, gel, cream, film, suppository or tablet), and a chemical that kills sperm.

How they work: These spermicidal preparations are inserted into the vagina before sexual intercourse. After insertion, the spermicide disperses and kills sperm before they pass through the cervix to the uterus.

How to use them: Contraceptive foam, gel, cream, film, suppositories or tablets are inserted into the vagina near the cervix. Spermicides must be reinserted each time the couple has intercourse. Foam, gel and cream are effective immediately. Film, suppositories and tablets are not fully effective until *15 minutes after insertion.* Spermicidal preparations remain effective no more than 1 hour after insertion. They also must be reinserted if more than 1 hour elapses between initial insertion and intercourse. All vaginal spermicides can be used alone, or with a diaphragm or latex condom for increased protection.

How and where to get them: Vaginal spermicides are available at supermarkets, drugstores, family planning clinics and online. A prescription is not required. There is no age limit for purchasing them.

Effectiveness and advantages: If used correctly every time a couple has sexual intercourse, spermicides alone are fairly effective at preventing pregnancy (82% with *perfect use* to 72% with *typical use*). When used *with a latex or polyurethane condom,* the combined method is very effective at preventing pregnancy, HIV and other STD. When used *with a diaphragm,* gels and creams are very effective at preventing pregnancy.

Risks and disadvantages: There are no health risks associated with using vaginal spermicides. Some people may have an allergic reaction or irritation. This can sometimes increase the risk of HIV and other STD transmission. If a reaction or irritation occurs, another brand may work better. Foam, gel or cream must be inserted right before having sexual intercourse; and film, suppositories and tablets must be inserted at least 15 minutes before intercourse. Spermicides need to be reapplied for each act of intercourse. ***When used alone, vaginal spermicides do not protect from HIV and other STD.***

Emergency Contraception

What it is: Emergency contraception (EC) is a method that reduces the risk of pregnancy after unprotected sex.

How it works: Emergency contraception prevents pregnancy primarily by stopping the egg from being released, so the sperm can't fertilize it.

How to use it: There are several different types of emergency contraception pills available in the United States. Depending on the type taken and the individual circumstances, a person may take one pill or several. EC works best when started as soon as possible after unprotected sex. It works best when started right away, but can be taken up to 5 days after sex. A copper IUD, inserted by a health care provider up to 5 days after unprotected sex, can also act as emergency contraception.

How and where to get it: Some kinds of pills are available from a pharmacist or at drugstores without a prescription. Other kinds require a prescription from a health care provider. A health care provider must insert the IUD.

Effectiveness and advantages: Taking EC as soon as possible or up to 5 days after unprotected sex can reduce the risk of pregnancy up to 89%. An IUD inserted within 5 days of unprotected intercourse reduces the risk for pregnancy by 99%.

Emergency contraception makes sense if a couple does not want to become pregnant and their regular birth control method was damaged, slipped out of place or wasn't used correctly. It can also be used to prevent pregnancy in cases of sexual assault.

Risks and disadvantages: Common side effects that can occur when taking EC pills include heavier menstrual bleeding, nausea, lower abdominal pain, fatigue, headache and dizziness. The IUD can cause increased menstrual bleeding, pain and/or cramping, as well as spotting between periods.

Some people do become pregnant or are already pregnant when they use emergency contraception. Studies have found no risk to a developing fetus from the use of EC pills. There is an increased risk of miscarriage from an IUD.

Emergency contraception should be viewed as a contingency measure. It is important for sexually active couples to practice a regular form of birth control. ***Emergency contraception provides no protection against HIV or other STD.***

Making a Difference! For Youth with Cognitive Impairments

DRUGS AND THEIR EFFECT ON SEXUAL RESPONSIBILITY

Reaching goals and dreams requires a person to be clear thinking, responsible and in control. Using alcohol and/or other drugs may prevent people from making the best decisions and, consequently, attaining their goals and dreams. Alcohol and other drugs alter thinking and impair judgment. This can lead to risky sexual behaviors. Below is a description of various drugs, what they look like and their effects.

ALCOHOL

(booze, brew, hair of the dog, hooch, juice, sauce, spirits)

Alcohol is the drug in beer, wine and liquor. When a person drinks alcohol, it goes straight from the stomach into the blood and then to the brain. Alcohol is a depressant and quickly changes the way the brain works.

What does it look like?

Alcohol is a colorless liquid that has a slight chemical odor. A standard drink has ½ ounce of pure alcohol. Each of the following alcoholic beverages is considered a standard drink:

- 12-ounce beer
- 10-ounce microbrew
- 8- to 9-ounce malt liquor
- 4 to 5 ounces of wine
- 1½ ounces of 80-proof liquor

What are its effects?

Drinking affects each person differently, depending on age, gender and body size, as well as how much and how fast a person drinks. How much food is in the person's stomach is also a factor. Only time will make a person sober. Drinking coffee, taking a shower, getting fresh air or vomiting will not get rid of the alcohol in a person's blood.

At the very early stages of drinking, alcohol can produce an enjoyable "buzz" effect. But when the blood alcohol level (BAL) reaches .05% to .06%, positive effects decrease and negative effects increase. Drinking too much on a single occasion impairs thinking and memory, slows reaction time, blurs vision, decreases inhibitions and can cause vomiting and passing out. At very high blood alcohol levels, breathing can stop, the heart can stop and death can occur from alcohol poisoning.

Chronic heavy drinking, or drinking too much over a long period of time, can cause serious health problems. These include the loss of memory and motor skills, heart damage, stroke, liver disease and an increased risk of certain cancers.

Some adults can choose to drink responsibly. They control how much they drink and stop before they drink too much. But some people become addicted to alcohol and can't control how much they drink. They can't stop before they drink too much and continue use despite personal harm or injury.

MARIJUANA

(pot, dope, grass, weed, Mary Jane, chronic, reefer, ganja, kaya, doobie)

Marijuana comes from the leaves of the hemp plant *cannabis sativa*. It can be eaten in certain foods or smoked. Medicinal and recreational use has been legalized in some places. But marijuana is illegal for anyone under age 21.

What does it look like?

Marijuana is a green or gray mixture of dried, shredded flowers and leaves.

What are its effects?

The effects vary from person to person depending on how strong the marijuana is, how it's taken and whether other drugs or alcohol are involved. At first, marijuana can make people feel relaxed, in a good mood and even silly. Users will likely experience dry mouth, rapid heartbeat, some loss of coordination, poor sense of balance and slower reaction times, along with intoxication. Blood vessels in the eyes will expand causing the red eye effect.

Marijuana in a person's system may impair short-term memory. This happens because all forms of marijuana contain THC (delta 9 tetrahydrocannabinol), the main active chemical in marijuana, which alters the way the brain works. After a few minutes, paranoia or anxiousness may set in, then intense hunger (a.k.a. the munchies). Finally, sleepiness may occur.

For some people, marijuana raises blood pressure slightly and can double the normal heart rate. This effect can be greater when other drugs are mixed with marijuana.

Marijuana can make people more likely to do things they might later regret. Like other drugs it impairs judgment and alters thinking. In addition, marijuana reduces coordination and concentration. It's harder to do many things, including sports, dancing, acting and studying.

Keep in mind that marijuana is illegal for anyone under 21. Using, holding, buying or selling it can get you suspended or expelled from school, and even a criminal record and jail time.

CRACK AND COCAINE

(coke, snow, blow, toot, nose candy, flake, the lady)

Cocaine is a powerful stimulant drug that comes from the leaves of the South American coca plant. Taking it makes people feel energetic and powerful at first, but then depressed, edgy and needing more.

What does it look like?

Cocaine is a white powder that people either snort or dissolve and inject with a needle. Crack is a form of cocaine that has been chemically altered and crystallized, so it can be smoked.

What are its effects?

At first, cocaine makes people feel energetic and powerful. As these feelings wear off, however, they quickly become depressed and edgy, and they experience intense craving for more.

Cocaine and crack are among the most addictive drugs available. Not only can these drugs harm the body, they can distort priorities to the point where all that matters is getting the next fix. Being high on cocaine or crack, or pursuing the next hit, often results in violence, car crashes, falls, burns and drownings.

People addicted to crack and cocaine often do risky things they later regret. They may spend all their money on these drugs and do any number of other things to support their habit, such as stealing from people they love, trading sex for money, selling drugs and getting involved in all kinds of other illegal activities. In their pursuit to feed the crack and cocaine addiction, users hurt the people around them and often end up alone.

INHALANTS

(all kinds of household goods, poppers, whippets, laughing gas, amyl nitrite, butyl nitrite, nitrous oxide, rush)

Inhalants are chemicals people sniff for a head rush. Usually, it's a product that's meant for something else, like gases, glue or cleaning products.

What are their effects?

People who use inhalants get a quick, giddy head rush. They are cheap and usually readily available, making them an easy choice for those who use them. Users feel slightly stimulated and uninhibited, but within a minute or two, a major headache comes on (the first indication that this is a bad idea). Hallucinations and numb hands and feet are often part of the package. Suffocation and sudden death can also occur, even during the first time a person uses these drugs.

HALLUCINOGENS

LSD (acid), psilocybin (mushrooms), mescaline

Hallucinogens change your thought processes, emotions and perceptions. The most popular are acid and mushrooms. LSD is the most potent hallucinogen.

What do they look like?

Acid usually comes in the form of a small piece of paper (blotter acid) that has been soaked in the drug. It also comes in small tablets called microdots or small squares of gelatin called window panes. When users place the acid on their tongue, the drug is absorbed and enters the blood stream. Mushrooms look like dried edible mushrooms, but they are not the same as the mushrooms you eat with foods like pizza. There are thousands of kinds of mushrooms. Hallucinogenic mushrooms are unique and contain a poison that makes you feel high.

What are their effects?

The effects of hallucinogens vary greatly—even unpredictably—depending on the dose, a person's mood, personality and surroundings. The effects usually begin 30–90 minutes after ingestion and can last up to 12 hours. The physical effects include dilated pupils, increased blood pressure, sweating, nausea, loss of appetite, sleeplessness, dry mouth and tremors. The major effects, though, are on the emotions and perceptions. Emotions while

 Making a Difference! For Youth with Cognitive Impairments

"tripping" may change frequently and vary widely—from fear and anxiety to euphoria. People's perceptions are also altered so that they lose their sense of time and direction and see distorted shapes and movements. Colors, sounds and smells may also be intensified. In some cases, a phenomenon known as synesthesia occurs, in which people report the ability to hear colors or see music.

When experiencing a "good trip," people feel a heightened sense of awareness. However, during a "bad trip," people may feel intense anxiety and a fear of dying or going insane. Furthermore, some people experience harmful psychological effects of the drug after the trip has ended. Psychological effects may persist for many years after and include severe mood swings, disordered thinking, loss of a sense of reality and visual problems. Some users experience flashbacks, which include hallucinations and other visual disturbances. These flashbacks may occur repeatedly for many years after they stop the drug, even after taking a hallucinogen only once.

DISSOCIATIVE DRUGS

PCP *(angel dust, ozone, wack, rocket fuel, supergrass)*
ketamine *(special K, vitamin K, cat valium)*
dextromethorphan *(DXM, robo)*

Dissociative drugs include PCP, ketamine and dextromethorphan. These drugs may create an out-of-body experience and detachment from the environment for the user. They affect the part of the brain that controls pain perception, memory, emotions and mood.

What do they look like?

PCP and ketamine both come in pill form or in powdered form to be snorted or smoked. Ketamine is odorless and tasteless, and has been used as a date rape drug because of this. Dextromethorphan is an ingredient in over-the-counter cough syrup. Users ingest many times the recommended dose for coughs when getting high on this drug.

What are their effects?

At low doses, PCP causes increased breathing, heart rate and blood pressure. At higher doses, it can cause dangerously rapid breathing, increased heart rate and increased blood pressure, as well as dizziness, nausea, blurry vision, decreased pain perception, muscle contractions and kidney damage. At extreme doses, PCP can lead to convulsions, coma and even death.

The psychological effects of **PCP** are unpredictable and may last from hours to days. Users experience detachment from reality, distortion of perceptions and hallucinations. It can also cause severe confusion, violence and suicide. PCP is addictive, and people may experience depression for years after stopping chronic use.

The effects of **ketamine** range from a dream-like state, euphoria, hallucinations and dissociation from one's body to complete sensory distortion and horrible feelings of death. At high doses, it can cause memory loss, high blood pressure and life-threatening problems with breathing.

The effects of **dextromethorphan** range from a mild effect and vision changes at low doses to a complete detachment from one's body at high doses.

Heroin

(smack, H, ska, junk)

Heroin is a highly addictive drug that comes from morphine. It produces a sense of euphoria that users constantly chase.

What does it look like?

It usually appears as white or brown powder, or as a black sticky paste. It can be injected, snorted or smoked.

What are its effects?

Short-term, heroin causes a sense of euphoria and clouded thinking that can lead to impaired decision making. This is followed by alternating wakeful and drowsy periods. Heroin causes depressed breathing and therefore overdose can be fatal. Injecting the drug increases a person's risk of contracting HIV and other blood-borne diseases.

 Making a Difference! For Youth with Cognitive Impairments

Methamphetamine

(speed, meth, chalk, ice, crystal, glass)

A highly addictive substance, closely related to amphetamine. It is toxic to the nervous system and has long-lasting effects. It is popular with teens as it is inexpensive and relatively easy to obtain.

What does it look like?

Methamphetamine can be in the form of a white powder that can be taken orally, snorted or injected. It could also be in the form of a rock or crystal that is heated and smoked.

What are its effects?

Methamphetamine increases energy, awake-time and physical activity. It increases the heart rate, blood pressure and body temperature. Long-term use can result in mood disorders, violent behavior, anxiety, confusion and insomnia. It can also result in severe dental problems. All users are at increased risk of contracting infectious diseases such as HIV and hepatitis.

MDMA

(ecstasy, XTC, E, Adam, hug, beans, love drug)

MDMA (ecstasy) is a popular drug among teens and young adults in the club and rave scenes. It has effects similar to both amphetamines (speed) and hallucinogens (LSD), such as increased energy, a dream-like state and euphoria.

What does it look like?

MDMA usually comes in a pill form. Pills come in a variety of colors and designs. It can also be snorted or injected.

What are its effects?

MDMA is a synthetic drug that has effects similar to both amphetamines (speed) and hallucinogens (LSD). The pleasurable effects of ecstasy include alertness, increased energy, euphoria, self-confidence and a feeling of closeness to others. Its effects last from 3 to 6 hours. The physical effects include nausea, muscle tension, teeth clenching, blurred vision, increased heart rate, increased blood pressure and increased body temperature. In high doses, body temperature can become dangerously high (called malignant hyperthermia), leading to muscle breakdown and kidney damage. Heart attacks, strokes or seizures may also occur in some people who use the drug.

New research is also finding that MDMA damages the area of the brain involved with memory, thought, mood and sleep. This damage can lead to depression, sleep problems, anxiety and paranoia. Furthermore, since this drug is synthetic, the actual content of the drug varies widely. Ecstasy pills may contain caffeine, dextromethorphan, heroin and mescaline in addition to MDMA. Accidental deaths have been reported among people who thought they were taking MDMA, but ingested another, more harmful drug instead.

TOBACCO

(bidi, butt, cigarette, cig, stoge, cancer stick, chew, dip, smoke)

Tobacco is an agricultural crop, most commonly used to make cigarettes. It is grown all over the world and supports a billion-dollar industry. The psychoactive ingredient is nicotine, a stimulant, but more than 4,000 other chemicals (2,000 of which are known to be poisonous) are present in cigarettes.

What does it look like?

Dried, cut-up leaves that are processed, dried and then either rolled and smoked or chewed.

What are its effects?

Nicotine, the main drug in tobacco, is highly addictive. It triggers complex biochemical and neurotransmitter disruptions. It elevates heart rate and blood pressure, constricts blood vessels, irritates lung tissue, and diminishes one's ability to taste and smell. Tobacco use will also lead to stained teeth, bad breath and premature face wrinkles. The health risks associated with tobacco are very serious and include cancer of the lungs, mouth, throat, esophagus and more; frequent feelings of cold; chronic bronchitis; emphysema; stroke; and heart disease.

PRESCRIPTION DRUGS

(opiates, stimulants, central nervous system depressants)

Prescription drug abuse means taking a prescription medication that is not prescribed for you, or taking it for reasons or in dosages other than as prescribed. Abuse of prescription drugs can produce serious health effects, including addiction. Commonly abused classes of prescription medications include opiates (for pain), central nervous system depressants (for anxiety and sleep disorders) and stimulants (for ADHD and narcolepsy).

What do they look like?

Prescription drugs like these most commonly come in pill form. The pills vary in color and shape depending on their type, brand and dosage and have different letters, numbers or symbols on them. For this reason, it is very easy to identify a pill that you may come across. However, when used recreationally, prescription pills can be crushed up into a powder, making identifying the substance more difficult. Additionally, prescription drugs can come in liquid form, to be taken orally.

What are their effects?

When taken properly, prescription drugs are effective and helpful to those who need them. However, when taken recreationally, they often have adverse and dangerous effects.

Opiates – Long-term use of opiates or central nervous system depressants can lead to physical dependence and addiction. Opiates can produce drowsiness and constipation and, depending on the amount taken, can depress breathing. Opiates act directly on the respiratory center in the brainstem, and if taken in excessive amounts, they can shut down breathing altogether and cause death.

Depressants – Central nervous system depressants slow down brain function. If combined with other medications that cause drowsiness or with alcohol, heart rate and respiration can slow down dangerously. Like opiates, they are extremely addictive.

Stimulants – Stimulants can increase blood pressure, heart rate and body temperature, and decrease sleep and appetite, which can lead to malnutrition and its consequences. Repeated use of stimulants can lead to feelings of hostility and paranoia. At high doses, they can lead to serious cardiovascular complications, including stroke. Addiction to stimulants is also a very real consideration for anyone taking them without medical supervision.

While on their own each of these drugs poses risks and health complications (especially when taken recreationally), when combined with other drugs or with alcohol, they are extremely dangerous. Mixing prescription pills with other drugs or alcohol can result in serious physical and mental problems and even death. Any prescription drug should be taken under the supervision of a licensed doctor.

Sources: National Clearninghouse for Alcohol and Drug Information. National Institute for Drug Abuse.

In summary, making proud and responsible choices will help you when you are faced with the many factors and influences that might impact your decisions about drugs.

Making a Difference! For Youth with Cognitive Impairments

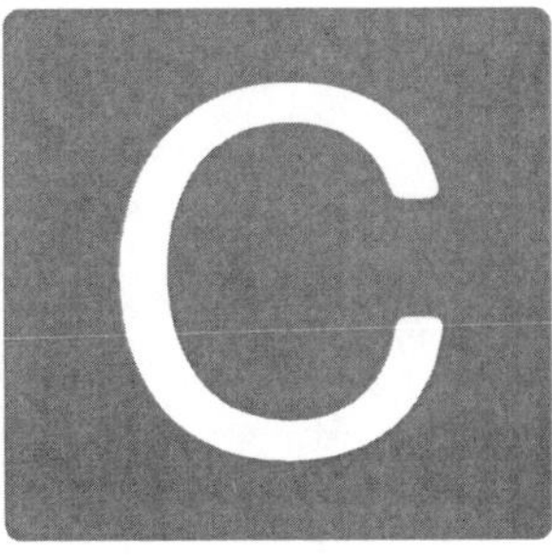

GROUP MANAGEMENT PROBLEMS AND STRATEGIES

Group management problems exist when one or more group members exhibit behaviors that interfere with, inhibit, deflect from or slow down the procedures or goals of the group. Some behaviors occur very rarely, others with greater frequency.

The following suggestions for dealing with group management problems will usually suffice, but even skilled facilitators must deal with new challenges that arise from time to time. Most methods for reducing group management problems are only a temporary bridge between initial participant resistance and the point in the process at which the participant regards participation to be useful, valuable and personally relevant. The following lists common management problems in adolescent groups and possible strategies for preventing and dealing with these problems.

TYPES OF GROUP MANAGEMENT PROBLEMS

INACTIVITY

Minimal Participation – Participants seldom volunteer a comment, provide only brief answers, and, in general, leave facilitators feeling as though they are struggling to keep the group on task.

Apathy – Apathy is a more extreme form of minimal participation. Almost everything the facilitator does to direct, enliven or activate the group is met with disinterest, lack of spontaneity and little if any progress toward group goals.

Falling Asleep – Participants may appear so uninvolved that they fall asleep. Before assuming this is due to lack of interest, inquire into the cause of the fatigue. Boredom, lack of sleep and physical illness are all possible reasons.

Excessive Restlessness – Participants fidget while sitting, rock their chairs, get up and pace, or display other nonverbal, verbal, gestural or postural signs of restlessness. Such behavior is often accompanied by digression, monopolizing or interrupting behavior.

ACTIVE RESISTANCE

Participation, but Not as Instructed – Participants are off target. They might be trying to roleplay, serve as co-actor, give accurate feedback, or engage in other tasks, but their own personal agendas or misperceptions interfere, and they wander off course to irrelevant topics.

Passive-Aggressive Isolation – Instead of participating as instructed, participants actively go off task and raise personal agendas. Passive-aggressive isolation is the purposeful, intentional withholding of appropriate participation and involvement.

Negativism – Participants signal overtly, by word and action, the wish to avoid participation in the group. They openly refuse to roleplay, provide feedback or complete assignments. They also might not come to sessions, come late to sessions or walk out in the middle of a session.

Making a Difference! For Youth with Cognitive Impairments

Disruptiveness – This includes displays of behaviors more extreme than negativism that are intended to interfere with the learning process. Examples include openly ridiculing the facilitator or other participants, and distracting nonverbal behaviors such as gestures, movements or noises.

HYPERACTIVITY

Digression – Participants act out repetitive and strongly motivated attempts to move away from the purposes and procedures. In some cases, the participants are feeling some emotion, such as anger, anxiety or despair, and are determined to express it. In other cases, activities set off associations, which the participants want to present and discuss. Digression is often characterized by jumping out of role in the roleplay. Rather than merely wandering off track, the participants drive the train off its intended course.

Monopolizing – This includes subtle and not so subtle efforts by participants to get more than a fair share of time during a session. Examples include long monologues, unnecessary requests to repeat roleplays, elaborate feedback and attention-seeking efforts.

Interruption – Interruption is similar to monopolizing, but more intrusive and insistent. Interruption involves breaking into a modeling display, roleplay or feedback period with comments, questions, suggestions, observations or other statements. An interruption might be assertive or angry, take the form of making faces or excessive humor or be presented benevolently as a helper.

COGNITIVE IMPAIRMENTS AND EMOTIONAL DISTURBANCE

Inability to Pay Attention – Closely related to excessive restlessness, the inability to pay attention often is a result of internal or external distractions that command a participant's attention. Inability to pay attention except for brief time spans also may be due to cognitive impairment.

Inability to Comprehend Concepts – The inability to understand key points and messages may be due to developmental disabilities, cognitive impairments, lack of experience or physical or emotional disorders. Failure to understand also can result from lack of clarity by the facilitator.

Bizarre Behavior – A number of such behaviors might include talking to oneself or inanimate objects, offering incoherent statements to the group, becoming angry for no apparent reason, hearing and responding to imaginary voices and exhibiting peculiar mannerisms. Such behavior not only pulls other participants off task but also can frighten them or make them highly anxious and is indicative of more serious mental health problems.

STRATEGIES FOR REDUCING GROUP MANAGEMENT PROBLEMS

SIMPLIFICATION METHODS

Reward Minimal Participant Accomplishment – Rather than responding positively to participants only when they enact a complete and accurate roleplay or other task, reward them for lesser, but still successful accomplishments, such as the correct portrayal of only one or two behavioral steps. In extreme examples, merely paying attention to someone else's roleplay could be the accomplishment.

Shorten the Task – Ask less of the participants by shortening the activity or roleplay.

Have the Participant Read a Prepared Script – This approach removes from participants the burden of figuring out what to say and eases getting in front of the group and acting out the skill. As with all simplification methods, using a prepared script should be a temporary device, used to move participants in the direction of roleplaying without assistance.

Have the Participant Play the Scripted Role First – Let participants who are uncomfortable with performing in front of their peers play the scripted roleplay first. This accustoms them to going before the group and speaking because the spotlight is mostly on someone else. This method should be used temporarily. Before moving on to the next skill, all participants should play the main role using the particular skill.

Making a Difference! For Youth with Cognitive Impairments

ELICITATION OF RESPONSE METHODS

Call for Volunteers – In the early stages, facilitators often elicit participation. The least directive way is calling for volunteers.

Introduce Topics for Discussion – Calling for volunteers in a highly apathetic group may yield no response. Under this circumstance, introduce discussion topics that appear especially relevant to the needs, concerns, aspirations and skill deficiencies of the particular participants.

Call on a Specific Participant – This is a more active and directive facilitator intervention. It is often useful to select a participant whose attentiveness, facial expression, eye contact or other nonverbal signal communicates potential involvement and interest.

Prompt and Coach Participants – The facilitator takes on the role of coach or prompter and feeds roleplay lines to a participant or carefully directs the group's discussion. The most direct way involves a facilitator standing behind the participant during a roleplay and whispering statements that represent each behavioral step for the participant to say out loud.

THREAT REDUCTION METHODS

Employ Additional Live Modeling by the Group Facilitator – The facilitator demonstrates a skill repeatedly. Such facilitator behavior makes it easier for the participants to get up and risk less-than-perfect performances in an effort to learn the skill. Such additional live modeling also proves useful to those participants who have difficulty roleplaying because of cognitive inadequacies.

Postpone the Participant's Roleplaying Until Last – A participant unwilling to participate is not required to roleplay until both the facilitator's live modeling and roleplaying by all other participants are completed. However, no participant should be excused completely from practicing the skill. To do so would run counter to the purpose of the group.

Provide the Participant with Direct Reassurance – In case of participant reluctance to roleplay, the following steps might be used as a guide for providing encouragement.

- **Step 1:** Offer resistant participants the opportunity to explain their reluctance to roleplay and listen nondefensively.

- **Step 2:** Express your understanding of the resistant participant's feelings.

- **Step 3:** If appropriate, respond that the participant's view is a viable alternative.

- **Step 4:** Present your own view in greater detail, with both supporting reasons and probable outcomes.

- **Step 5:** Express the appropriateness of delaying a resolution.

- **Step 6:** Urge the participant to try to roleplay the given behavioral steps.

METHODS FOR TERMINATING INAPPROPRIATE RESPONSES

Urge Participants to Remain on Task – Bring the participants back on track gently, but firmly. Do this by pointing out to participants what they are doing incorrectly and reminding them of the target behaviors.

Ignore Participant Behavior – Inappropriate behaviors can be terminated by ignoring them. This withdrawal of reinforcement, which leads to the extinction process, is best applied to behaviors that the group can tolerate while still remaining on task as the process is taking place. Deal with behaviors that are more disruptive or dangerous to the group's functioning more directly.

Interrupt Ongoing Participant Behavior – Interrupt ongoing participant behavior when other methods fail. Do it firmly, unequivocally, and with the clear message that the group has its tasks. It might require removing a participant from the group for a period of time.

Making a Difference! For Youth with Cognitive Impairments

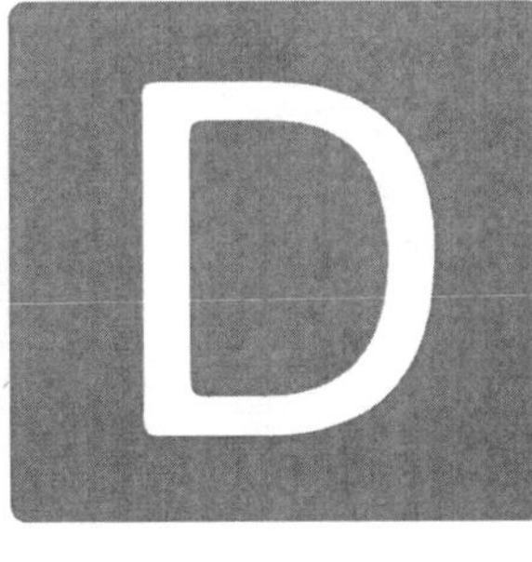

SUPPORTING A TRAUMA-INFORMED APPROACH TO SEXUALITY EDUCATION

Trauma is prevalent among youth in this country, and the need to address trauma in youth programming is increasingly clear.[1] Trauma occurs when individuals are exposed to harmful or threatening events that overwhelm their ability to cope in the moment or in the future.[2] These include experiences of physical, emotional or sexual abuse, neglect, caregiver substance use or mental illness, family instability, assault and community violence.[3] Not all children and youth are the same, and they may respond differently in the face of these exposures based on their subjective experience of the event(s), their age, their history of exposure and available resources and supports.[2,4]

Advances in neuroscience show that intense or ongoing exposures to traumatic events, without protective factors, alter the body's stress response system—affecting a young person's cognitive, social and emotional development.[3] In the classroom setting, these physiological changes can manifest as problems or challenges with learning, paying attention, regulating emotions, showing self-control and developing trusting relationships.[2] In severe cases, young people may exhibit symptoms of post-traumatic stress disorder (PTSD) or child traumatic stress. Potentially traumatic experiences are also part of the constellation of risk factors associated with early sexual initiation,[5] more sexual partners,[6,7] unprotected sex[7] and teen pregnancy,[7,8] as well as poorer mental health and substance use.[9]

Schools, youth-serving organizations and educators play an important role in recognizing and responding to trauma, as well as promoting healing and resilience for trauma survivors. A trauma-informed approach: (1) realizes the widespread impact of trauma and understands potential paths for recovery; (2) recognizes the signs and symptoms of trauma in students, staff and families; (3) responds by fully integrating knowledge about trauma into policies, procedures and practices; and (4) resists re-traumatization by avoiding practices that inadvertently create stressful or toxic environments.[1]

Specific practices educators, youth workers, schools and youth-serving organizations can implement to cultivate trauma-informed sexuality education include the following:

- Provide training to staff so that they understand the effects of trauma and know how to recognize and respond to it appropriately.[1,10,11]

- Create a culture of safety so that both staff and participating youth feel physically and psychologically safe.[1,10] This includes establishing clear agreements around privacy, respect for self and others and appropriate behavior for the group setting.

- Build and maintain trust and transparency in relationships.[1] For sexuality education, it is especially important to inform youth and parents about the educator's obligation to report incidents in which young people disclose abuse or the intent to harm themselves or others.

- Create a culture of empowerment that recognizes people's individual strengths, resiliency and ability to heal from past trauma.[1,10]

- Recognize that trauma can arise from power differences due to culture, gender and sexual orientation.[1,10] Use inclusive language that empowers diverse populations. Avoid stigmatizing particular groups of youth or reinforcing limiting stereotypes.

- Facilitate open conversations. Regardless of past experiences, all youth benefit from conversations that allow them to feel positive about their bodies, negotiate relationships and determine when they are ready to engage in safe, consensual sexual activity.[10]

- Avoid judgment or attaching shame to past experiences or current sexual behaviors, particularly teen parenting and sexually transmitted infections.[10]

- Be aware that some students' behavior problems that arise in the group setting may stem from past trauma. Adopt disciplinary policies that focus on restoring relationships and integrating offending students back into the school and community. Traditional disciplinary policies that focus on punishment often aggravate the sense of rejection felt by someone with a history of trauma.[11]

In addition, many educators and youth workers who work with traumatized youth also are vulnerable to the effects of trauma. This is often referred to as compassion fatigue or secondary traumatic stress. Educators can help avoid compassion fatigue by becoming aware of the signs (such as increased irritability with youth, difficulty planning lessons and activities, feeling numb or detached or intrusive feelings about a student's trauma), asking for support from colleagues, seeking help to heal from their own personal traumas and engaging in self-care by setting boundaries, eating well, exercising and taking a break when needed.[2]

Making a Difference! For Youth with Cognitive Impairments

1 SAMHSA. 2014. SAMHSA's *Concept of trauma and guidance for a trauma-informed approach.*

2 National Child Traumatic Stress Network Schools Committee. 2008. Child trauma toolkit for educators. Los Angeles, CA & Durham, NC: National Center for Child Traumatic Stress.

3 Harvard Center for the Developing Child. Key concepts: Toxic stress. Available at: http://developingchild.harvard.edu/index.php/key_concepts/toxic_stress_response.

4 Lieberman, A. F., & Knorr, K. 2007. The impact of trauma: A developmental framework for infancy and early childhood. *Pediatric Annals,* 36: 209.

5 Black, M. M., Oberlander, S.E., Lewis, T., et al. 2009. Sexual intercourse among adolescents maltreated before age 12: A prospective investigation. *Pediatrics,* 124: 941–949.

6 Felitti, V. J., & Anda, R. F. 2014. The lifelong effects of adverse childhood experiences. *Child Maltreatment,* Vol. 2., 4 ed., 203–216. Saint Louis: STM Learning, Inc.

7 Homma, Y., Wang, N., Saewyc, E., & Kishor, N. 2012. The relationship between sexual abuse and risky sexual behavior among adolescent boys: A meta-analysis. *Journal of Adolescent Health,* 51: 18–24.

8 Hillis, S. D., Anda, R. F., Dube, S. R., et al. 2004. The association between adverse childhood experiences and adolescent pregnancy, long-term psychosocial consequences, and fetal death. *Pediatrics,* 113: 320–327.

9 Shonkoff, J. P., & Garner, A. S.; the Committee on Psychosocial Aspects of Child and Family Health; Committee on Early Childhood, Adoption and Dependent Care; and Section on Developmental and Behavioral Pediatrics; et al. 2011. The lifelong effects of early childhood adversity and toxic stress. *Pediatrics,* 129: e232–246.

10 Fava, N. M., & Bay-Cheng, L. Y. 2013. Trauma-informed sexuality education: Recognising the rights and resilience of youth. *Sex Education,* 13: 383–394.

11 Oelhlberg. B. 2009. Why schools need to be trauma informed. *Trauma and Loss: Research and Interventions,* Fall/Winter: 1–4.

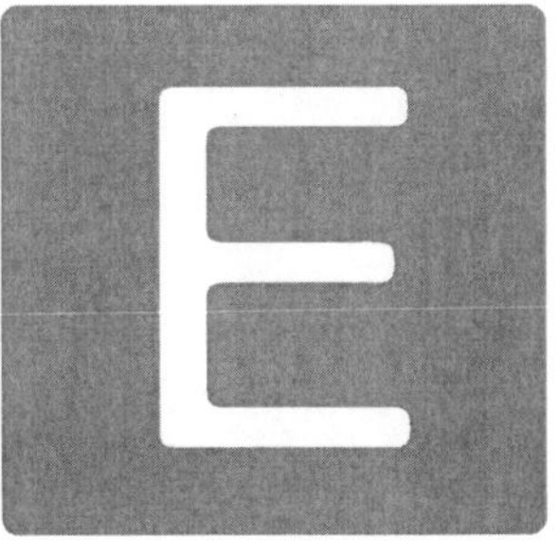

ANSWERS TO COMMON QUESTIONS ASKED BY ADOLESCENTS

QUESTIONS ABOUT HIV/AIDS

1. Does AIDS affect people of all races?

- Yes. Anyone, regardless of race, can acquire HIV if that individual participates in risky sexual or needle-sharing behaviors with an infected person.

2. What causes AIDS?

- AIDS is the end result of an infection caused by a virus called the human immunodeficiency virus.

3. Can people of all ages get HIV?

- Yes. People of all ages can get the virus if they are exposed to it through risky behaviors. Even children can get HIV. The majority of infected children acquired the virus from an infected mother during pregnancy or childbirth. Others acquired the virus during breastfeeding. Some children became infected from blood transfusions before blood supplies were routinely screened for HIV.

4. Is HIV infection like other diseases?

- HIV infection is not like communicable diseases such as a cold, flu or measles that can be passed through casual contact, including sneezing, coughing or sharing eating utensils. No cases have been established where HIV was passed by those means.

5. Can you carry the virus and not develop AIDS?

- Yes. Worldwide there are people who are infected with HIV and have not developed AIDS. Many people who are HIV positive do not know they are infected. People with HIV can transmit it to others even if they don't have any symptoms.

6. How does HIV break down the immune system?

- Scientists know that the virus destroys the white blood cells of the immune system. White blood cells consist of T-cells and B-cells and protect a person from disease. Some T-cells, also called helper cells, or CD-4 cells, help the B-cells produce antibodies against invading disease-causing organisms. When HIV enters the body, it infects/destroys the helper (CD-4) cells. When you lose CD-4 cells, your immune system breaks down and it becomes difficult to fight infections/diseases.

7. How contagious is HIV?

- In comparison to other communicable diseases, HIV infection is much less contagious than germs of the common cold, flu, measles and tuberculosis. These diseases can spread through the air, whereas HIV is spread only through infected body fluids.

8. Can you get HIV from casual contact?

- No one should be afraid of becoming infected through casual contact. Transmission of the virus takes place during behaviors in which certain bodily fluids are exchanged, including semen, vaginal secretions, rectal fluids, blood or breast milk.

  People can, for example, work with others, attend school and public events, eat at restaurants and be around people with HIV without the fear of getting HIV. People who are caring for another family member who has HIV or AIDS are also not at increased risk for contracting the virus. Children attending school with another student who is HIV positive are not at increased risk for becoming infected.

9. Can you get HIV from kissing?

- No. You cannot get HIV from a kiss on the cheek or a closed-mouth kiss. There are extremely rare cases of HIV being transmitted via deep "French" kissing, but in each case, infected blood was exchanged due to bleeding gums or sores in the mouth. Because of this remote risk, it is recommended that individuals who are HIV positive avoid deep, open-mouth "French" kissing with a non-infected partner, as there is a potential risk of transferring infected blood.

Making a Difference! For Youth with Cognitive Impairments

10. **What can an individual do to keep from getting HIV?**

- People can reduce their risk of contracting HIV by practicing responsible behavior around sexual expression and drug use. Responsible sexual precautions include: (1) sexual abstinence, (2) sexual fidelity, (3) avoiding exchange of body fluids by using a condom, and (4) avoiding sexual partners who have engaged in risky behaviors. These precautions can also help prevent the contraction of other STDs. Responsible behavior regarding drug use includes abstaining from using drugs at the most, and avoiding sharing needles and syringes at the very least.

11. **Can HIV/AIDS be cured?**

- There is no cure for HIV, but anti-retroviral treatments (ART) can be started while the person still feels healthy. With ART medicines, people with HIV can lead longer and healthier lives than ever before. The most common treatments limit the ability of the virus to reproduce. They help protect the immune system and improve the chances of staying healthy. Pregnant women with HIV can take medicines to greatly reduce the baby's risk of having HIV.

12. **Is there a vaccine for HIV?**

- No. Scientists are working to develop a vaccine, but a solution appears to be many years away.

13. **Should a student with HIV be allowed in school?**

- Yes. A student living with HIV or AIDS poses no risk to other students. However, there may be times when the person might not be able to attend school because of illness.

14. **Should people with HIV be banned from public events, schools and jobs?**

- No. Since HIV cannot be passed by casual contact, there is no reason why a person living with HIV or AIDS should be kept from being a participating member of a community.

15. **Can HIV be transmitted during oral sex?**

- Absolutely. Whenever there is vaginal, anal or oral sex between two people and one is HIV positive, the virus may be transmitted to the uninfected person. The vagina, anus and mouth are lined with sensitive tissues called mucous membranes, which can come in contact with blood, semen, vaginal secretions or rectal fluids during all types of intercourse. The virus can enter an uninfected person's bloodstream through tiny tears in the mucous membranes that occurred during sex or that were there beforehand. These tears can be very small, existing without any pain or visible blood to act as a warning sign.

The safest option is to practice sexual abstinence. If that's not your choice, then knowing your partner well enough to communicate openly with each other about diseases and precautions lessens your risk. Couples should use a new latex or polyurethane/polyisoprene condom every time they have sex, including oral sex. For oral sex on a woman, dental dams can be used. These are available in many drugstores or can be made by cutting a non-lubricated condom lengthwise and opening it up to cover the vulva. Partners can also get tested for STDs, including HIV, before they begin having sex with each other.

16. Is it possible to have HIV and not have any visible symptoms? If so, how can I know if a partner is infected?

- Yes, it is possible for a person to have HIV and not have symptoms. One way to find out if your partner is infected is by asking. The foundation of love and responsible sex is good communication. An open and honest discussion with someone you know and trust will probably result in the truth. But remember, people might not know that they have HIV or another STD. If you are concerned that your partner might have HIV or another STD, you and your partner may want to be tested just to be sure.

17. How effective are condoms in preventing the transmission of HIV and other STDs?

- If used properly, latex condoms are highly effective against most STDs, including HIV. Proper use of condoms means:

  » Using latex or polyurethane/polyisoprene condoms, not lambskin.

  » Using fresh condoms that have been stored in a cool, dark place (not a wallet or a glove compartment).

  » Handling the condoms carefully, avoiding damage from rings and fingernails and keeping them rolled up or in the package until you are ready to use them.

  » Putting the condom on as soon as erection is achieved.

  » Leaving some room at the tip of the condom when it is put on.

  » When a lubricant is desired, using only water-based lubricants such as K-Y Jelly®.

18. Isn't AIDS a gay disease?

- No. AIDS, a result of HIV infection, is caused by a virus (HIV). Anyone can get HIV through the exchange of blood, semen, vaginal or rectal fluids with an infected

Making a Difference! For Youth with Cognitive Impairments

person. Like anyone else, men who have sex with men are at higher risk only if they engage in activities that include the exchange of these fluids.

19. Why are injection drug users at high risk for getting HIV?

- Injection drug users who share needles and works with others have an increased risk of getting HIV because drops of blood from one person can cling to the needle or works. When a person is shooting up, infected blood can pass HIV directly into the bloodstream of another person.

20. Are Hispanics and African Americans more likely to develop AIDS than other ethnic groups?

- Although HIV infection affects us all, the number of AIDS cases among Hispanics and African Americans is proportionately higher than that of the general population. The reasons for this difference are linked to socioeconomic factors (e.g., level of education, income, access to health care, etc.) and not to racial factors.

21. If I am HIV positive or am at risk for HIV infection, whom should I tell?

- Telling someone you have HIV isn't easy. Consider telling your doctors, dentist and dental hygienist, and be sure to tell your sex partners (past, present and future). If you share needles and syringes, also tell these partners.

22. Can I get HIV from kissing on the cheek?

- Kissing on the cheek is very safe. Even if the person kissing you has HIV, your skin is a good protector.

23. Can I get infected with HIV by someone who performs oral sex on me?

- It is unlikely that you would get HIV if an infected person performed oral sex on you. However, if the person receiving oral sex has HIV or AIDS, the person performing oral sex can get it.

24. Is vaginal sex dangerous? If I have only vaginal sex, can I get infected with HIV?

- HIV is caused by a virus, and if a person has the virus, vaginal sex puts that person's partner at risk for HIV infection. Many women have gotten the virus from their infected male partners during vaginal sex. Many men have been infected by their female partners during vaginal sex as well. Couples should use condoms every time they have sex if either partner is infected or unsure of his or her HIV status. Though condoms sometimes break, they greatly lower the chances of HIV transmission from one partner to another.

Appendix E // FAQ/GLOSSARY

25. How can vaginal sex cause HIV infection in women?

- A woman can get HIV from vaginal sex if her partner is infected. The walls of the vagina are surrounded by blood vessels. HIV infected semen can enter the woman's body, usually through tiny cuts and tears in the walls of the vagina that the woman might not even know about.

26. Can I get HIV from anal sex?

- Yes. If either partner is infected with HIV, the other partner can be infected during anal sex. Generally, the person receiving the semen is at greater risk of getting HIV because the lining of the rectum is thin and contains many blood vessels. However, the person who inserts the penis is also at risk if the partner is infected because HIV can enter through sores or abrasions on the penis.

27. If I just fool around, can I get HIV?

- It depends what you do. You can get HIV, the virus that causes AIDS, if the blood, semen, vaginal secretions or rectal fluid of an infected person enters your bloodstream in any way.

28. What sexual activities are safe?

- Safer sexual activities include:
  - » No sex—oral, anal or vaginal
  - » Sex between two mutually monogamous, uninfected partners who do not share needles or syringes with anyone
  - » Body rubbing/massaging, mutual masturbation (*Caution:* safe against HIV and some other STDs only as long as bodily fluids are not exchanged. Some STDs [herpes, HPV] can be passed by unprotected skin-to-skin contact.)
  - » Massaging one's own genitals, self-masturbation
  - » Kissing and other activities that do not include touching the penis, vagina or rectum

29. Can a woman get HIV from having sex with a man? Can a man get HIV from having sex with a woman?

- Yes. Either a woman or a man can become infected during oral, vaginal or anal sex if the partner is HIV positive.

 Making a Difference! For Youth with Cognitive Impairments

30. **Can lesbians get HIV?**

   - Yes, but cases of woman-to-woman transmission of HIV where unprotected sex was the only risk factor are extremely rare. Like anyone else infected with HIV, any infected woman who has sex with other women can infect her partner(s) during sex if certain bodily fluids are exchanged.

31. **If I pick my sexual partner carefully, am I safe?**

   - You can't tell by looking or asking questions whether or not someone has HIV. The only way to be sure is for a person to be tested.

32. **Are condoms effective? How safe are they? I've heard they fail 10 percent of the time. Is that true?**

   - Latex or polyurethane/polyisoprene condoms help protect you from the transmission of HIV and other disease agents. They greatly reduce your risk of infection if used properly. Condom failures usually result from improper use.

33. **How can someone get infected with HIV from a needle?**

   - Because the virus can be spread through blood-to-blood contact, the person using a contaminated needle or syringe is at high risk of getting HIV. A contaminated needle can carry the virus directly into the bloodstream. This includes needles used for body piercing and tattooing as well.

34. **My teammates and I use needles to take steroids. I share needles only with my friends. Can I get HIV?**

   - Yes. If any of your friends or teammates has HIV and you share needles and syringes, you could become infected. Remember, it isn't just the type of drug that the needle is used for; it is the behavior that creates the risk. Also, you can't tell by the way someone looks whether that person has HIV or not.

35. **What drugs are associated with getting HIV?**

   - The use of alcohol, cocaine, crack, heroin and amphetamines is associated with the transmission of HIV. These drugs affect people's judgment and may lead to high-risk activities such as having unprotected sex or sharing needles for any purpose.

36. Why is crack associated with HIV?

- Crack is a form of cocaine that is smoked. People who use it have a higher risk of becoming infected with HIV because of activities associated with crack culture and because it reduces a person's decision-making skills.

37. Can I get HIV from someone's saliva?

- There are no documented cases of saliva transmitting HIV. While there is a theoretical possibility of spreading HIV by saliva, research suggests that it is highly unlikely.

38. What if someone with HIV bites me? Will I get AIDS?

- It's rare, but in 1997, someone in the United States became infected from a bite by an HIV-infected person. The potential for transmission exists if the skin is broken and blood is exchanged.

39. Can I get HIV from the tears of someone with AIDS?

- No. There is no evidence that anyone in the United States has become infected with the virus from touching the tears of an infected person.

QUESTIONS ABOUT SEXUALLY TRANSMITTED DISEASES

40. I'm a teenager; I'm not at risk for getting an STD, right?

- Wrong. Young people ages 15 to 24 account for nearly half of all new cases of STD each year.* There are other STDs out there besides HIV, and they are on the rise among teens. These include chlamydia, gonorrhea, syphilis, herpes and human papillomavirus (HPV), which causes genital warts and can lead to cervical cancer.

41. Can you get an STD from a public restroom?

- This is not very likely. Most STDs are only transmitted during sexual contact, either by skin-to-skin contact or through body fluid exchange. Crabs, or pubic lice, may be transmitted through sexual contact, sleeping in infected bedding and sharing infected clothing. Lice cannot survive away from the human body for longer than 24 hours, so contracting pubic lice from a toilet seat is unlikely.

* Centers for Disease Control and Prevention. 2015. STDs in Adolescents and Young Adults. From www.cdc.gov/stds/stats14/adol.htm. Accessed 1/5/16.

 Making a Difference! For Youth with Cognitive Impairments

42. Can I get HIV or another STD from getting a tattoo or through body piercing?

- There can be a risk for HIV or another blood-borne infection (such as hepatitis B or C) if the instruments used for piercing or tattooing are not properly sterilized or disinfected between clients. Any instrument used to pierce or cut the skin should be used only once and thrown away, or thoroughly cleaned and sterilized before it is used again. Ask the staff at the parlor about their equipment. They will show you what precautions they use.

43. Can I get an STD from kissing?

- This is possible but not very common. If your partner's mouth is infected with an STD, then he or she may be able to pass that infection to your mouth during a kiss. Fever blisters and cold sores can be passed through a kiss if your partner is infected. Blood-borne infections such as HIV or hepatitis B or C can be passed through kissing only if there is an exchange of infected blood. If your partner has an infection in his or her genital area, then kissing on the mouth will not transmit the infection.

44. Can I get an STD from oral sex?

- Yes. During oral sex, there is skin-to-skin contact and bodily fluid exchange, so it is important to use barrier methods such as unlubricated condoms or dental dams to protect you during oral sex.

45. Why don't teens who are having sex protect themselves from STDs?

- They may:

  » Be embarrassed about buying or getting condoms.

  » Feel peer/date pressure.

  » Use alcohol and drugs, which affects their judgment.

  » Have a lack of knowledge.

  » Believe using birth control pills is enough protection.

  » Be embarrassed about asking questions.

  » Not think about it ahead of time.

46. How do I get tested for an STD?

- There are different tests for each of the different STDs. Some STDs are hard to test for if you do not have any symptoms. Some STDs can be identified through a simple blood test or a urine test; others can be detected only through culturing body

fluid from the penis, vagina or open sore on the body. If you go in for testing, it is
important to ask your health care provider which tests will be done and which will
not. Sometimes, weeks or months need to pass to give your body enough time to
develop antibodies that will show up in a test.

47. Where do I go to get tested?

- Your local health department, community clinic, private doctor or Planned
  Parenthood are all good locations to check out for STD testing. The CDC National HIV
  STD Testing website lets you look up free or low-cost clinics in your area that do STD
  testing: gettested.cdc.gov.

48. What's the difference between confidential and anonymous testing?

- All medical care that you receive should be confidential. This means that the
  information you discuss with your health care providers must stay in your files at
  the clinic or doctor's office and not be released to anyone without your permission.
  Anonymous testing is when your name is not associated with the test or the results
  in any way. You are given a number or code word to identify yourself during testing
  and when receiving results.

49. Do my parents have to find out if I get tested for STDs and HIV?

- No, clinics will see you without your parents' permission. If you are concerned about
  this, call the clinic before you go. Ask if you need to bring your parent along for
  permission and what information the clinic will share with them. This way you know
  what to expect ahead of time.

50. What are the common symptoms of STDs?

- STDs can cause physical symptoms such as bumps or sores on the skin, discharge,
  pain or burning during urination (peeing) or symptoms like the flu. Some STDs do
  not cause any symptoms at all.

51. Can I have an STD and not know it?

- Yes. STDs can take weeks, months or even years before symptoms show. Some
  people never develop any symptoms for some STDs. However, STDs can still be
  transmitted whether or not the person has symptoms.

 Making a Difference! For Youth with Cognitive Impairments

52. How do I know if my partner is infected?

- The simple answer is that you may not know unless your partner knows and tells you or gets tested and shows you the results.

QUESTIONS ABOUT PREGNANCY

53. Can you get pregnant by kissing?

- No. The only way a woman can get pregnant is if sperm cells enter her vagina and fertilize one of her egg cells. This usually happens during vaginal sex, but can also happen if a man ejaculates near the entrance to the vagina, but not inside it, or if sperm is introduced into the vagina by hand.

54. Can a boy get a girl pregnant if he has not had a wet dream?

- Yes. A boy can get a girl pregnant whenever he is able to have an ejaculation. Even if a boy has never had a wet dream, his testicles may be producing sperm.

55. If a girl misses her period, is she definitely pregnant?

- Certainly not. When girls first start having periods they often have irregular cycles and may even skip a month from time to time. However, if a girl has had sexual intercourse and she misses a period, she could be pregnant. She should take a pregnancy test and see a doctor right away.

56. Can a girl get pregnant if she has sex standing up?

- Yes. Sperm does not care what position you are in. Any time semen comes in contact with the vagina a girl may get pregnant. There are no exceptions to that rule. There are no safe positions or safe times for having sex without risking pregnancy.

57. Can a girl get pregnant the first time she has vaginal sex?

- Yes, if she has started ovulating and there is an egg present, it can be fertilized by a sperm. A girl may ovulate before she has had her first period, so not menstruating yet is not a guarantee of not getting pregnant.

58. Can a girl get pregnant from swallowing semen?

- No. The only way a girl can get pregnant is if sperm cells enter her vagina, usually during sexual intercourse, and fertilize one of her egg cells.

59. Can douching after intercourse prevent pregnancy?

- No. Douching will not prevent pregnancy; it only pushes the sperm up the vagina increasing the chance of pregnancy. Douching may also cause irritation and lead to infection.

60. Is withdrawal (pulling the penis out of the vagina before ejaculation) a good way to avoid pregnancy?

- No. This is the way many teenage girls get pregnant. Withdrawal requires a great deal of self-control. Interrupting sexual intercourse can be very difficult for people "caught up in the moment." Also, sperm sometimes may be present in pre-ejaculate fluid, and pulling the penis out just before ejaculation will not keep these sperm from entering the partner's body.

61. Can Vaseline prevent pregnancy?

- No. Vaseline does not contain anything to kill sperm, so it is not a contraceptive. Also, Vaseline collects bacteria, is thick and greasy, and is hard to wash off.

Making a Difference! For Youth with Cognitive Impairments

GLOSSARY

ABSTINENCE: Not having oral, vaginal and anal sex or doing any other behaviors, such as skin-to-skin genital contact or touching, that can cause a pregnancy or pass an STD.

ACNE: Small, swollen spots or pimples on the skin on a person's face, neck, back or chest. Acne is common during puberty due to hormones and because a person's skin starts to make more oil.

ACQUIRED IMMUNODEFICIENCY SYNDROME (AIDS): a serious disease of the immune system caused by a virus called HIV.

AIDS: See acquired immunodeficiency syndrome

ANAL SEX (ALSO ANAL INTERCOURSE): Sexual activity in which a penis is put in the anus.

ANUS: The opening between a person's buttocks where solid waste (poop) leaves the body.

BEHAVIOR: Something a person does.

BIRTH CONTROL: Something that prevents pregnancy (the pill, IUD, condoms).

BISEXUAL: Being romantically or sexually attracted to people of both the same and different sex.

BODY FLUIDS: Liquids made in and by the body, such as tears, saliva, sweat, blood, vaginal fluid, semen, rectal fluids and breast milk. Some diseases can be passed when someone comes in contact with the blood or other body fluids of someone who has the disease.

BODY HAIR: Hair on the body, such as on the legs, arms, chest and face. Body hair starts to grow during puberty.

BOUNDARY: A limit that defines OK behavior; a line a person does not want to cross; a rule about what should not be done.

BREASTS: Two soft parts on the chest that produce milk when a woman has a baby; breasts develop during puberty.

CASUAL CONTACT: Day-to-day social contact, such as a hug or kiss on the cheek, shaking hands, or using a telephone, toilet or swimming pool. Colds and flu can be spread this way, but not HIV.

CERVIX: The opening to the uterus from the vagina. The cervix can get wider so that a baby can be born.

CLITORIS: A very sensitive sex organ located in front of the opening to the vagina.

COMMUNICATION: The act of sharing your ideas, thoughts and feelings with someone else. Clear and open communication can help create trust, respect and equality in healthy relationships.

CONDOM: A thin rubber covering that fits over an erect penis during sex in order to prevent a pregnancy or the spread of diseases. Can be made out of different materials (latex, polyurethane, polyisoprene or lamb intestines). Also see female condom

CONSENT: Permission or agreement; when both people clearly and freely agree to engage in a behavior.

CONSEQUENCES: Things that happen due to an action, choice or behavior; results or outcomes.

CONTAMINATED NEEDLES: Needles that have been used by someone with an infection or disease (HIV, hepatitis B). Needles that are not clean can spread diseases.

CUDDLING: To hold someone or something in your arms while lying or sitting close together as a sign of affection.

CURIOUS: Wanting to learn or know more about something.

DATING: Doing an activity with someone you have or might want to have a romantic relationship with; spending time and doing activities with a romantic partner.

DECISION: A choice you make about something after thinking it through.

DELAY: To wait until later to do something; to put off doing something until later.

DISEASE: An illness that affects a person; a condition that prevents the body or mind from being healthy and working properly.

DRY KISSING: To touch lips without mouth-to-mouth or tongue contact; examples include social kissing and kissing on the cheek.

EGG: A reproductive cell made in the ovaries. An egg is released during ovulation, and then travels down the fallopian tubes to the uterus. If the egg is fertilized by a sperm, it will implant in the uterus and begin to grow during pregnancy.

EJACULATE: To release semen from the penis during orgasm.

EJACULATION: The release of semen from the penis during orgasm.

EQUALITY: The state of being equal or the same for each person. For example, having the same rights or social standing.

Making a Difference! For Youth with Cognitive Impairments

ESTROGEN: A hormone made by the ovaries that causes the female reproductive system to develop and function.

FALLOPIAN TUBE: Two tubes that go from the ovaries to the uterus; an egg travels through these tubes to get to the uterus.

FERTILIZED EGG: An egg that has been joined by a sperm and can now implant in the uterus to begin a pregnancy.

FRENCH KISS: A kiss done with mouths open and tongues touching. (See open-mouth kiss)

FUTURE: The period of time or events that will come after the present time (today).

GAY: A term for people who are romantically and sexually attracted to someone of the same sex. Most often used to refer to males who are attracted to other males and whose sex partners are men.

GENDER: A person's sense of being male or female. Gender roles are ideas or expectations about how a male or female should behave that can come from a person's family, culture, friends and society. Gender identity refers to the inner way people see and feel themselves as being male or female and may or may not match the way others see them. Gender expression is how people express their gender to the outside world such as in how they dress or the things they like to do.

GENITAL CONTACT: Touching the external reproductive organs of a partner. Some diseases can be spread through skin- to-skin contact of the genitals.

GENITALS: The sexual and reproductive organs on the outside of the body. Examples include the vulva, penis, and scrotum.

GOAL: Something you are trying to do or achieve.

HETEROSEXUAL: Being romantically or sexually attracted to people of a different sex. Also referred to as straight.

HIV: See human immunodeficiency virus.

HIPS: The part of the body between the waist and legs on each side. During puberty, a girl's hips get wider.

HORMONES: A natural substance made in the body that cause changes in how our bodies grow and develop.

HUMAN IMMUNODEFICIENCY VIRUS (HIV): The virus that causes AIDS. It attacks and damages the immune system so that a person can no longer fight off illnesses.

I-STATEMENT: A way of sharing thoughts and feelings without blaming another person. I-statements focus on the speaker's feelings and help the other person understand the speaker's point of view. Examples: "I feel…", "I need…" "I would like…" instead of "You did…" or "You are…."

IMMUNE SYSTEM: The body's system of defense against disease; made up of special cells, proteins in the blood and other body fluids.

IMMUNE: Protected from a disease.

INFECTION: A disease caused by germs that enter the body; can be caused by bacteria or a virus.

INTERCOURSE: Sexual activity between two people; a type of contact involving (1) putting a penis into a vagina (vaginal intercourse); (2) using the mouth to touch the genitals of another person (oral sex); or (3) putting a penis into the anus of another person (anal sex).

LABIA: The folds of skin at the outer part of a woman's sexual organs to protect the opening to the urethra and vagina.

LESBIAN: A term for females who are romantically or sexually attracted to other females and whose sexual partners are women.

LIMIT: A point beyond which a person is not allowed to or chooses not to go.

MASTURBATION: Touching one's own genitals for sexual pleasure.

MENSTRUATION: The flow of blood and tissue out of the vagina from the uterus; occurs about once a month after puberty. Also called having a period.

MENSTRUAL CYCLE: The time from the first day of one period to the first day of the next period. During the menstrual cycle, the lining of the uterus grows, an egg is released by the ovaries, and the lining of the uterus leaves the body through the vagina if the egg has not been fertilized.

MONOGAMOUS: Having sex with only one other person. This can help protect people from HIV and other STDs, but only if both people test negative for infections before they have sex, and then agree to have sex only with each other.

MUSCLES: Body tissue that contracts to produce movement.

MUTUAL MASTURBATION: When two people touch each other's genitals for sexual pleasure or masturbate in front of each other.

OBSTACLE: Something that gets in the way or makes it hard to do something.

Making a Difference! For Youth with Cognitive Impairments

OPEN COMMUNICATION: Open and honest sharing of thoughts and feelings between people; an important part of healthy relationships. Ways to support open communication include talking face to face, listening to each other's point of view, using I-statements and being respectful.

OPEN-MOUTH KISS: A kiss that involves tongue-to-tongue contact. (See French kiss.)

ORAL SEX (ORAL INTERCOURSE): Sexual activity that involves using the mouth to touch the genitals of another person.

ORGASM: The point during sexual activity when sexual pleasure is strongest; often when ejaculation occurs.

OVARIES: Reproductive organs that store and release eggs and make hormones, including estrogen.

OVUM: Another term for the egg stored and released by the ovaries.

PEER: A person in the same age group or social group.

PENIS: The male sexual organ through which semen and urine leave the body. The penis gets erect during sexual arousal.

PERIOD: The flow of blood and tissue out of the vagina from the uterus; occurs about once a month after puberty. Also called menstruation.

PERMISSION: Agreement or approval to do something. Asking permission means asking if you can or cannot do something.

PITUITARY GLAND: A small organ in the brain that produces hormones and influences growth and development (puberty).

PREGNANCY: The time during which the fertilized egg grows from an embryo to a fetus in the uterus. It lasts about 40 weeks (or about 9 months) from the time the fertilized egg implants in the uterus to the birth of a baby.

PRESSURE: Force or efforts from others to get you to do something; a feeling of worry or anxiety that you need to agree or go along with someone else's ideas or actions. Peer pressure is the feeling that you must do the same things as other people of your age and social group in order to be liked or respected by them.

PRIVATE: A place where there is only one person. A place in which you are usually alone or other people are prevented from entering.

PROUD: Feeling happy or pleased because of something you have done, something you own, someone you know or are related to; feeling satisfied and worthy.

PUBERTY: The stage of life when the reproductive system matures and a young person starts to change into an adult and becomes able to have children. It is if normal for puberty to begin any time between ages 9 and 16. A person's feelings, moods and emotions about self, family and others change too.

PUBIC BONE: One of the bones that makes up the pelvis.

PUBIC HAIR: Hair that grows around the external genitals during puberty.

PUBLIC: A place where there is more than one person. Places where you are likely to see other people or other people are with you or could join you.

RESPECT: Admiration for and treating someone or something as good, valuable or important.

RESPONSIBLE: Able to be trusted to do what is right or take care of something; doing the things that are expected or required.

RISK BEHAVIOR: An activity that puts a person at increased risk for getting HIV and other STD. (Examples: sexual activity with multiple partners without a barrier, sharing needles)

ROLEPLAY: An activity in which people practice skills by acting out a sample situation.

SALIVA: The liquid (spit) made in your mouth that keeps your mouth moist and makes it easier to swallow food.

SCHOLARSHIP: An amount of money given to a student to help pay for that student's education.

SCROTUM: The loose sac of skin that holds the testicles; it helps keep the testicles at the right temperature for making sperm.

SEMEN: Milky-white fluid containing sperm that is ejaculated from the penis during orgasm.

SEX (SEXUAL INTERCOURSE): A type of sexual contact involving: (1) putting a penis into a vagina (vaginal intercourse); (2) using the mouth to touch the genitals of another person (oral sex); or (3) putting of a penis into the anus of another person (anal sex).

SEX: The label of male or female assigned to a person at birth.

SEXUAL ATTRACTION: A feeling of desire for sexual contact or sexual excitement toward another person.

SEXUAL FANTASY: A thought, idea, or daydream that causes sexual excitement.

SEXUAL ORIENTATION: Describes a person's feelings of sexual attraction toward others, including to which gender a person is sexually attracted. Some common sexual orientations include gay, lesbian, straight and bisexual.

SEXUALITY: All the aspects of human behavior having to do with sex and gender. Includes sexual function and behavior, but also includes choices around sex, feelings of being male or female and communication about sex.

SEXUALLY ACTIVE: Engaging in sexual behaviors that can put a person at risk of pregnancy, HIV and other STDS.

SPERM: The reproductive cell made in the testicles that can fertilize an egg.

SEXUALLY TRANSMITTED DISEASE (STD): Infection that's passed from one person to another during vaginal, anal or oral sex, or during sexual skin-to-skin contact. Also called sexually transmitted infection.

SEXUALLY TRANSMITTED INFECTION (STI): Infection that's passed from one person to another during vaginal, anal, or oral sex, or sexual skin-to-skin contact. Commonly known as sexually transmitted disease.

STRAIGHT: Being romantically or sexually attracted to people of a different sex.

SWEAT: A clear liquid produced from the skin when a person is physically active, hot or nervous.

SYNDROME: A group of related symptoms or diseases/disorders.

TAMPON: A firm, disposable roll of absorbent cotton or other fiber that goes inside the vagina to absorb the blood and tissue shed during menstruation (a period).

TESTICLES: Reproductive organs that produce sperm and the hormone testosterone. Also referred to as *testes*.

TESTOSTERONE: A hormone made in the testicles that causes the female reproductive system to develop and function.

TOUCHING: To use a hand, fingers or parts of the body to feel someone or something.

TRANSGENDER: A general term used to describe people whose gender expression/gender identity are different than the sex they were assigned at birth.

TRANSMITTED: To cause a virus or disease to be given to others. Some diseases can be spread during sexual contact with an infected person.

TRUST: To believe that someone or something is reliable, good or honest; to have confidence in someone or something; to feel safe with another person in a relationship.

URETHRA: The tube that empties the bladder and carries urine (pee) out of the body. The urethra also carries semen out of the penis during ejaculation.

URINARY OPENING: The opening to the urethra where urine (pee) leaves the body.

URINE: Waste liquid that collects in the bladder before leaving the body.

UTERUS: The pear-shaped reproductive organ where a pregnancy develops.

VAGINA: A muscular tunnel that goes from the outside of the body to the uterus. It provides a way for menstrual fluid to leave the body, receives a penis during vaginal intercourse and provides a way for a baby to be born.

VAGINAL OPENING: The end of or opening to the vagina where menstrual fluid leaves the body and where a baby comes out during childbirth. It is located in the vulva below the urinary opening.

VAGINAL SEX (ALSO CALLED VAGINAL INTERCOURSE): Sexual activity in which a penis enters a vagina. Also called "vaginal intercourse" or "penis-in-vagina sex."

VALUE: A strong belief about what is worthwhile, important or right; someone or something's worth or importance; to hold something as important, useful or worth something.

VIRUS: A disease agent that enters the cells of the body to reproduce, often destroying these cells. For example, HIV is the virus that causes AIDS.

VOICE: The sounds made with the mouth and throat when speaking or singing. The voice may change as a person goes through puberty.

VULVA: The region on the outside of the female body that includes the clitoris, urethral opening, labia and vaginal opening.

WET KISS: See open-mouth kiss. A kiss made with the mouths open and the tongues touching.

WOMB: The uterus.

 Making a Difference! For Youth with Cognitive Impairments